the complete
book of
water
healing

Ancient Healing Secrets:
Practical Herbal Remedies from Around the World That Work Today

The Complete Guide to Natural Sleep

Deadly Medical Mysteries: How They Were Solved

Dian Dincin Buchman's The Natural Way to Get Well and Stay Well

How to Be Safe in Any Emergency Book: The Family Take Charge Book

Making Dreams Come True:
Solving Life Problems by Directing Your Dream-Time

Natural Healing Secrets

Superimmunity for Kids (with Leo Galland, M.D.)

the complete book of water healing

Using the Earth's most essential resource to cure illness, promote health, and soothe and restore body, mind, and spirit

Dian Dincin Buchman, Ph.D.

Contemporary Books

Chicago   New York   San Francisco   Lisbon   London   Madrid   Mexico City
Milan   New Delhi   San Juan   Seoul   Singapore   Sydney   Toronto

Library of Congress Cataloging-in-Publication Data

Buchman, Dian Dincin.
    The complete book of water healing : Dian Dincin Buchman.
        p.   cm.
    Includes index.
    ISBN 0-658-01378-5
    1. Hydrotherapy.   I. Title.

   RM811.B778   2001
   616.8'53—dc21   2001029544

Contemporary Books

A Division of The **McGraw-Hill** *Companies*

1 2 3 4 5 6 7 8 9 0   AGM/AGM   0 9 8 7 6 5 4 3 2 1

ISBN 0-658-01378-5

This book was set in Adobe Caslon and Trade Gothic by Carolyn Wendt
Printed and bound by Quebecor—Martinsburg

Cover design by Lisa LeConte
Cover photo by Pete Turner, Inc. © Imagebank
Interior design by Laurie Young

McGraw-Hill books are available at special quantity discounts to use as premiums and sales promotions, or for use in corporate training programs. For more information, please write to the Director of Special Sales, Professional Publishing, McGraw-Hill, Two Penn Plaza, New York, NY 10121-2298. Or contact your local bookstore.

The purpose of this book is to educate. It is sold with the understanding that the publisher and author shall have neither liability nor responsibility for any injury caused or alleged to be caused directly or indirectly by the information contained in this book. While every effort has been made to ensure its accuracy, the book's contents should not be construed as medical advice. Each person's health needs are unique. To obtain recommendations appropriate to . your particular situation, please consult a qualified health-care provider.

This book is printed on acid-free paper.

This book is dedicated to four generations
of my adventurous and courageous family:
Hannah Pearl Meyerwitz, my grandmother;
Renee Meyerwitz Dincin, my mother;
Caitlin Dincin Kraft Buchman, my daughter;
and especially Dylan Tomasso Dincin Kraft and
Oriana Chiara Dincin Kraft,
my amazing grandchildren.

contents

preface   xiii

introduction   xvii

part 1   1
Using Water to Heal

   Water Is Holistic Medicine   4
   How Water Works in Your Body   7
   Forms of Water   8
   Clean Water   10
   Water and Weight Loss   14

part 2   19
Water Healing Techniques

MEDICAL USES OF WATER   19
DRINKING WATER   35
ICE   41
COMPRESSES   47
BATHS   67
FOOTBATHS   85
HAND BATHS   95
HERB AND MEDICATED BATHS   99
SHAMPOO   115
PACKS   119

SHOWERS   129
STEAM   141
TONIC TECHNIQUES   145
PERSPIRATION INDUCTION   149
CLAY   153

part 3   157
Water Healing for Common Ailments

Abscess   157
Acne   158
Arthritis   159
Asthma   162
Back (Lower Back Problems)   164
Bad Breath   165
Bedwetting   166
Body Odor   167
Bursitis   168
Canker Sores   169
Carpal Tunnel Syndrome   169
Chronic Fatigue Syndrome   170
Colds   171
Cold Sores   173
Constipation   174
Contact Lens Problems   175
Coughs   175
Cramps   177
Depression   177
Diabetes   178
Diarrhea   180
Digestive Problems   182
Dry Mouth   184
Ear Problems   185
Eczema   187
Elimination   188
Fatigue   189
Fever   190

Flabby Muscles	192
Flu	193
Food Poisoning	196
Foot Problems	197
Frostbite	201
Gallbladder Symptoms	202
Gout	202
Gum Problems	203
Hay Fever	204
Headaches	205
Heart Problems	208
Heat Reactions	211
Hemorrhoids	213
Herpes Simplex	214
Hiccups	215
High Blood Pressure	216
Hernia (Hiatus Hernia)	217
Incontinence	217
Indigestion	220
Infection	222
Inflammation	224
Inflammatory Bowel Disease	226
Insect Bites	227
Irritable Bowel Syndrome	227
Itching	230
Jet Lag	232
Kidney Stones	232
Laryngitis	234
Leg Cramps	235
Mouth Sores	236
Nervousness	237
Neuralgia	237
Neuritis	238
Nosebleed	238
Pain	239
Periodontal Disease	240
Pleurisy	241

Pneumonia   242
Poison Ivy, Poison Oak, Poison Sumac   244
Psoriasis   245
Ringworm   247
Rosacea   247
Scars   248
Sciatica   249
Shingles   250
Sinus Infection   251
Sore Throat   254
Stiff Neck   256
Tapeworm   256
Temporomandibular Disorders   257
Tonsillitis   257
Ulcers   259
Urination   260

part 4   261
Water Healing for Men, Women, and Children

WATER HEALING FOR MEN   261
Fertility and Hot Baths   261
Prostate Problems   261
Sexual Lassitude   264
Spermatorrhea (Involuntary Discharge of Semen)   265
Testicular Inflammation (Orchitis)   266
WATER HEALING FOR WOMEN   267
Breast Abscess (Mastitis)   267
Inflamed Breasts   268
Childbirth   269
Cystitis   270
Menopause   271
Menstrual Problems   272
Pregnancy   277
Other Pelvic Area Problems   278
Vaginal Problems   279

WATER HEALING FOR CHILDREN   283
    Bad-Tasting Medicine   283
    Bedwetting   283
    Boils   283
    Chickenpox   283
    Colic   284
    Cold Sores   284
    Congestion   285
    Constipation   285
    Convulsions   285
    Crying Spell   285
    Cuts   286
    Diarrhea   286
    Diphtheria   286
    Dizziness   287
    Ear Infections   287
    Eczema   288
    Eruptions   288
    German Measles   288
    Hernia   289
    Heat Reaction   289
    Mastoiditis   289
    Measles   290
    Mumps   292
    Nightmare Zap   293
    Scarlet Fever   293
    Sleeplessness   294
    Stomachaches   294
    Strengthening for Children   294
    Teething   295

part 5   297
Water Healing, Sports, and Exercise

    Exercise Recovery   300
    Achilles Tendon   300

contents

Ankle Injuries 300
Arch Spasm 302
Arm Injuries 302
Blisters 306
Bruises 306
Callus 311
Chest Strain (Pectoral Strain) 312
Eye Injuries 313
Finger Injuries 314
Foot Injuries 315
Genital Injuries 316
Hand Injuries 318
Jockstrap Itch 319
Knee Injuries 319
Muscles 323
Shin Injuries 326
Shoulder Injuries 327
Sprain and Swelling 331
Stitch 332
Tendinitis 333
Thigh Injuries 334
Toe Injuries 336

resources 339

index 347

preface

I write this preface for the posthumous publication of my mother, Dian Dincin Buchman's, *The Complete Book of Water Healing*, with great pride. My mother was both an innovator and a searcher, a pioneer on issues of natural health long before these issues were mainstream or fashionable. She came from a long line of inquiring, courageous, and adventuresome people.

My mother's grandmother Hannah Pearl started a natural cosmetics line in Romania, leaving her children and husband alone in the countryside to pursue her dreams. Romanian Gypsies took care of my mother's mother, Renee, during this period, and the Gypsies left an indelible impression on her, including their use of many household foods and plants as natural remedies. Renee walked miles to and from a Baron de Hirsch school for Jewish girls every day. There she learned not only Romanian, French, German, Latin, and Hebrew but the many insights into the natural world and healing that she passed along to her children, including my mother, her daughter Dian.

My mother's father, Herman Dincin, came to the United States alone from Russia at sixteen to pursue his great dream of becoming a doctor, a healer. His tuition stolen, he studied pharmacy at Columbia University instead. However, he lost faith in "the drug business" after a few years of pharmaceutical practice. Herman Dincin then became a chiropractor in an age when this was both intellectually and physically a daring act. Many of his colleagues were put in jail for "practicing medicine without a license." One had to be deeply committed and passionate about the practice of chiropractic in those days, in the 1920s.

As for my mother and her own search, in her own era she became an expert day by day quite by accident. As a young mother, she found no answers for my childhood eczema (except cortisone) and began research that quickly took her through traditional medical books, to nutrition, and back to some of the most simple and ancient ways of curing simple, and simply cured dis-ease.

She began writing on issues of natural beauty, tapping many of Hannah Pearl's secrets in *Feed Your Face,* published in 1973 in England, and retitled for American publication as *The Complete Herbal Guide to Natural Health and Beauty.* She was always a believer in folk traditions and oral traditions, a lover of simple histories. Her inquiring mind and delight in research earned her a Ph.D. in health science with a special area of concentration in the chemical properties of water and water's physiological action on the body. That research led to the original edition of this book, published first in 1979 as *The Complete Book of Water Therapy,* revised extensively in 1994, and completely rewritten in late 1999 for this millennium edition. She wrote over fifteen books in all, most on different natural health topics. Her books' common themes are the simplicity and power of natural healing, with emphasis on ancient and traditional folk remedies, and plain old common sense.

Water therapy was one of my mother's great loves precisely because of water's simplicity. Water has a profoundly important part in supporting life, but its power as a healing agent is often forgotten. How can something so ubiquitous be so incredibly effective, and affordable for all? This moved my mother. In an age when medicine is trying to find its way back to its best traditions, and patients are taking more responsibility for their own health again, this revised and updated classic on water healing comes at a potent moment. Water. Simple, powerful, and profound. Words to describe water, words to describe my mother's work, and words to describe my mother.

If you enjoy this book and share what you find useful in it, you too will continue this enduring folk tradition and chain, and that would please my mother very much.

CAITLIN DINCIN KRAFT BUCHMAN

introduction

grew up in a family that truly enjoyed doing most things naturally. We used water—especially cold water—as our primary health aid, and many other water treatments for the prevention and remedy of minor health problems. In our daily arsenal we used hot and cold compresses, showers, short "dunks," long baths, as well as dozens of other water techniques, and we always knew how to quickly overcome fatigue, sore throats, and colds. In fact, with our knowledge of water, herbs, and exercise we rarely needed "heavy" doctoring. We drowned incipient colds with determined water drinking, detoxifying baths, and perspiration-inducing herbal teas. We also used many kinds of off-the-shelf home products, as well as everyday foods, our garden flowers, and herbs in various forms, in our home ministrations. Because we had constant success with these treatments, we never hesitated to use them for emergency first aid for cuts, bumps, sprains, burns, delayed or protracted menstrual periods, or the ordinary health problems that occur daily.

During my childhood all these things had seemed so effortless that as I grew up I was bewildered to discover that other people used complicated medicines to get the same effects that we achieved with only water. I was stunned when I discovered that my neighbors and friends requested antibiotics for even the most minor ailment.

To my present chagrin, at one point in my late teens and early twenties, I just didn't want to feel—or be—different from all these other people, and I joined them. It wasn't until I became less energetic, and my husband and child seemed to be ill more often, that I decided to retrieve all my inherited knowledge of natural healing, and also to investigate other forms of nondrug health approaches. My family's remarkable range of water therapies proved to be one of the exciting answers in my quest for knowledge.

In her girlhood, my maternal grandmother had a short, but extraordinary, contact with Romanian Gypsies. She taught me many native and Gypsy remedies that used plants and household foods. But it was the Dincins, my father's family, who taught us water therapy concepts. Many of my father's uncles and other relatives were "old-fashioned" physicians who believed in the body's natural ability to heal itself when properly stimulated. They were, and are, a very adventurous group. One had traveled to Worishaven, Bavaria, to observe how the great nineteenth-century master Sebastian Kneipp conducted his "water cure" therapies. He also studied with Dr. Wilhelm Winternitz, the Austrian scientist who researched the direct and indirect nerve reactions from water. This great-uncle then joined with other pioneers and investigated the action of various states of water on the human body and, together with other forward-thinking physicians and lay healers, utilized water in their private and hospital practice.

My father's uncle, Dr. Herman Dincin, worked with all the early, great exponents of American hydrotherapy. Among them was the outstanding Dr. Simon Baruch, the physician who actually brought hydrotherapy to America. At first this system was received indifferently, but later it was used by some of the great internists, including Sir William Osler.

Several of these clinically minded physician-hydrotherapists wrote papers or books on their experiences. Among those I and my father's family are deeply indebted to include Dr. William Dieffenbach, professor of bacteriology at New York Medical College and Hospital for Women, and later professor of hydrotherapy at Flower Hospital; the great health reformer, Dr. J. H. Kellogg, who advised lay people in *The Uses of Water in Health and Disease;* various physicians for religious groups that stressed nondrug medicine, among them Dr. George Knapp Abbott, dean of faculty, professor of physiology, and superintendent of Loma Linda Hospital in California; and Dr. R. Lincoln Graham, the inventor of the graham cracker, who also wrote *Water in Disease and in Health,* and who achieved astonishing cures with water.

Although Uncle Herman was first a family doctor and then an endocrinologist, his secret passion was plain old water therapy. Our family had always used the simple double throat compress (a cold-water compress followed by a wool bandage to keep out air), and various other cold-water packs and compresses. Uncle Herman taught me about cold-water food splashes and cold-water treading to increase disease resistance, and the value of the circulation-inducing and inexpensive pickup: the coarse salt rubdown before a bath. He explained to me how and why these and innumerable other water therapy techniques worked on the body.

Anyone can learn to use water as therapy—for pleasure and to provide better health and more energy.

You will never regret learning the water therapy concepts. Because they are so easy to do and can be put into effect the minute you start to feel ill, they will make your life less complicated and ultimately give you more and better control of your health.

part 1
Using Water to Heal

*W*ater therapy is as old as humanity, and it is ironic that such a natural, effective medicine has to be rediscovered in each era. One of the first written mentions of the use of water as medicine is from the temples of the Greek god of medicine, Asclepius. Hippocrates used water as a beverage to reduce fever and to treat many diseases. He also stressed the value of using various types of baths, each with a different temperature, as a therapeutic tool to combat illness.

Later, the ancient Roman physicians Galen and Celsus also advocated specific baths as an integral part of their remedies. A series of cold baths are known to have cured the Roman Emperor Augustus of a baffling disease that had resisted all other remedies, and thereafter cold baths were much in vogue in Rome.

Almost every warm-climate civilization has at some time used baths for therapeutic reasons as well as for pleasant social interaction. There is an interesting medical footnote on the great Persian physician Rhazes, who was the first to comment on the difference between measles and smallpox. Rhazes wrote on the action of perspiration in forcing the eruptions to quickly emerge. This concept is very important in water therapy and has been known and used by physicians in India, Turkey, Russia, and Finland, as well as by the medicine men of the American Indians.

Throughout history there are indications that water was used as a remedy in controlling high fevers, but the remedy was so simple that its use waned as other modes of treatment were introduced. It is interesting to note that during the eighteenth century there was a great revival of the use of water as medicine among some Italian, German, and English clergymen. The dedicated Scottish physician and surgeon Dr. James Currier wrote an important book, *The Effects of Water, Cold and Warm, as a Remedy in Fever and Other Diseases,* in which he detailed his clinical use of cold-water drinking and dousing to reduce high fevers, particularly those of typhoid and smallpox, and his use of cold water for its internally stimulating and reactive powers.

Currier wrote his first book in 1797. However, it was not until the early nineteenth century that Vincent Preissnitz, a Silesian farmer, laid the foundation of modern water therapy. Vincent was only a teenager when he first become interested in water's healing powers. He had mangled his fingers and, as he watched with amazement, a neighbor showed him how to use continuous wet, cold compresses to cure and restore the function of his injured fingers. Shortly after this episode, Vincent was loading hay into a cart on a hill when the horses bolted and the heavy cart rolled over his body. Preissnitz remembered the lesson of his fingers. He daringly forced his caved-in ribs into a more natural position, and again tried cold compresses to relieve his pain. The combination of rest, copious water drinking, and wet cold wrappings worked beyond his wildest dreams. He fully recovered, and water therapy was "invented" once again.

History is studded with such isolated medical successes, but what is really extraordinary is that this teenage farmer took his own experience with a therapy and developed it into a whole therapeutic system. Preissnitz's cure was so spectacular that he immediately won the respect and interest of his fellow villagers. Because he had so many varied health problems to work with, Preissnitz was able to experiment with folk remedies, concepts that strangers brought to him from other lands, and his own variations. And since he was tenacious and analytical, he developed many new techniques for using water: single- or double-compress packs, dousings, full and partial immersions, and, of course, those famous cold "douches"—streams of water that we call showers.

Word soon spread of this extraordinary farmer who could perform miracles with water. Hundreds of sick people came from all parts of the Austro-Hungarian Empire. Under the direction of Preissnitz, each house in the village of Grafenberg was transformed into a miniature spa. Although his system won many followers, it also provoked great controversy among practicing physicians who eventually took Preissnitz to court. He not only won his case, but the leading physician of the empire, Baron Turkeim, came to observe his methods and reported to the emperor that they worked. Thereafter, Preissnitz was under the protection of the Crown, and visitors came to him from every land.

One of these visitors, English disciple Dr. Erasmus Wilson, noted that Preissnitz was able to devise these simple, yet intricate techniques "because his mind wasn't cluttered with the medical impossibilities of such an achievement."

Preissnitz did not write down his procedures—rather, they were written up by literate men or physicians who came to observe his system. He had a startling impact on English, German, and some Scandinavian, as well as American, disciples, but it wasn't until Sebastian Kneipp that water therapy became truly international.

Kneipp was born in 1821, in Bavaria, a few years after Preissnitz. He was a weak and frail youngster who was determined from early childhood to become a priest. However, repeated illnesses interfered with his studies and activities. During one of his many long convalescences, he chanced to read a pamphlet (we do not know whether it was one by a religious colleague or one about Preissnitz) that discussed the use of cold water to strengthen the body and make it disease-resistant. The concept electrified him. Although it was the heart of the Bavarian winter, he went to the river and plunged in. Determined to strengthen himself, he repeated this icy plunge every day, and in a short time he became markedly stronger. He developed extraordinary stamina, vigor, and strength, which he maintained through a long and active life as a priest. Cold water and water therapy made him the renowned Charles Atlas of his day.

Kneipp shortened some of Preissnitz's techniques, and also developed strengthening concepts of walking either in cold water or on wet grass. We owe the next set of innovative hydrotherapy procedures to his clinical activities.

Kneipp was also a practicing herbalist, and he combined many herbal therapies with the water techniques. Among his most important contributions was the use of such inexpensive herbs as hayflower or oatstraw for detoxification purposes. He experimented with healing procedures for a great many diseases, and was particularly active in helping to heal children. He developed the wet "nightshirt," dipped either in salt water or hayflower water, and this was one of the keystones of his treatment for children's diseases.

After Kneipp, many prominent English, German, and American scientists investigated the therapeutic action of water on the body. I am indebted to these scientists, physicians, and lay persons who continuously observed and noted the clinical action of water on children and adults who recovered from acute or chronic conditions as a result of hydrotherapy.

WATER IS HOLISTIC MEDICINE

Water is a natural medicine that benefits the entire body. It can be used in a variety of versatile, no-side-effect ways to help control and cure acute conditions—everything from diarrhea to a cold to migraine headaches—as well as chronic bad health. It can also be used as a disease deterrent and superior health safeguard. The vast number of techniques and therapeutic uses that involve water are collectively known as water therapy, or hydrotherapy. Water therapy, in turn, is a part of a general approach to good health known as holistic medicine.

Holistic medicine has several elements: a three-part approach to total health that stresses the interaction of the mind, body, and nutrition; a desire to always investigate the general cause, as well as the specific symptom, affecting the body; a need to take responsibility for your own health; a sense of partnership with a caring health practitioner.

In holistic, nondrug medicine, one of the important aims is to overcome sudden or chronic energy blocks and to restore the normal flow of internal energy to the affected part, or to the entire body. Water therapy is a remarkable reenergizer, which can be used for first aid as well as many other everyday problems. In restoring the energy flow, water therapy helps the body to heal itself and prevents many other health problems from occurring. It is therefore in the first line of health defense, and it should be considered an important tool in self-care and self-caring medicine.

Water can and should be part of your daily health routine. When you take a warm bath to relax or a short cold shower to stimulate your tired body, you are unconsciously using the techniques of water therapy. I start each day with two personal therapies: I drink two glasses of cold water about an hour before breakfast, and I march for a few minutes in a shallow cold footbath. The drinking overcomes an inherited tendency for sluggish peristalsis, and the cold-water treading boosts my energy and is a long-range body strengthener.

Every person who has ever lived on earth has used water for survival, for without drinking water we would die. But because we normally drink water only to quench our thirst and as a solvent for our food, we tend to ignore its manifold health benefits and the fact that water is needed internally by every functioning cell and organ.

I've discovered that just drinking a lot of plain, cold water will help to revitalize me during sluggish periods. Physicians and chiropractors often find that weak muscle response, particularly if all the muscles are responding in the same way, may be due to minor dehydration. One glass of drinking water sometimes overcomes this strange, total body weakness. Drinking water also can help reduce a high fever, stimulate one organ to interact with another, and cleanse internally by eliminating unwanted material from the system.

What makes treatment with water so unique is that it is always as available as the nearest running water. Moreover, water therapy is painless, and hundreds of different health problems can be treated immediately, naturally, and at little or no cost. Water therapy can stop a cold before it starts, help overcome a sore throat, generate energy, relieve pain, vanquish nervousness, help induce sleep, awaken a fogged brain, reestablish internal good health, and even help us to feel sexier; in short, it can restore and tone the body.

What is exceptional about water therapy is that it works with each person's own nature. Water therapy acts in a positive way and never destroys valuable internal flora, nor does it deplete the energy of internal organs. Water therapy creates circulation and overcomes sluggishness; it also unblocks an energy barrier so that the body can function in a freer and normal fashion. By acting to detoxify—that is, to rid the body of any accumulated poisons or toxins that may be the start of disease, or linger after a disease—water therapy increases our body's natural defense mechanisms.

Dr. William Kellogg, an early twentieth-century advocate of natural foods and natural healing, noted that in perfect health each part of the body receives its due share of blood. Water can equalize the circulation of the blood, control and equalize temperature, relieve pain, stimulate a sluggish or inactive organ, remove foreign or toxic material from the system, and stimulate or soothe the entire nervous system.

Another reason for using the techniques of water therapy is related to the behavior of bacteria in the body. Scientists have discovered that genetic material can mutate from one bacterium to another, making them far stronger and more virulent than prior generations of similar bacteria. Dr. Stanley Falkow, of the University of Washington, calls these "jumping genes," and it is his gloomy prediction that more and more bacteria will leap into a new stage. This has happened to *Haemophilus influenzae,* the causative pathogen in some cases of bronchitis, meningitis, pneumonia, and sinusitis. Penicillin used to be able to destroy this bacterium, but now doctors are dismayed to find many patients no longer respond to penicillin treatment.

Scientists have also discovered the alarming fact that other bacteria have become antibiotic-resistant, the way many insects achieved DDT-resistance. More and more virulent strains of certain deadly bacteria are emerging, for example, those that cause Legionnaires' disease, which is now turning up in all parts of the country and which has been classified as an unknown strain of pneumonia. Another example is a new form of typhoid now unresponsive to the antibiotic chloramphenicol. In Mexico, a recent epidemic decimated 14,000 patients before physicians could successfully switch to another antibiotic, in this case, ampicillin.

There is no doubt that antibiotics are successful, but there is also no doubt that the persistent use of antibiotics poses its own dangers. In the natural evolutionary process, any organism will develop successful mutations that are increasingly resistant to the medicines that previously combated them. In the widely hailed British documentary *The Overworked Miracle,* an American scientist, Dr. Sidney Ross, chief of microbiology at Children's Hospital in Washington, D.C., forecast that this overuse of antibiotics all over the world has created new and more deadly diseases. In Dr. Ross's words: "I think we will be looking back fifty years hence, at this as being somewhat of a golden era . . . we may be reverting back to the Middle Ages, as far as antibiotic therapy goes!"

If Dr. Ross's statement is true, and we will have increasing trouble controlling many lethal diseases that are now under control, it will be necessary to reacquire all the forgotten wisdom of nondrug healing. Water therapy—as a serious and effective alternative to toxic drug medicine—is an excellent place to start.

It is possible that water therapy is partially effective because it is so enjoyable. Some scientists say we feel better in water because the sea is our true ancestral home. Others liken the feeling of relaxation in water to the memory of the amniotic fluid we were suspended in before birth.

Of the many different water therapies, none is more rewarding than the bath for fun and relaxation. What parent can forget the look of pleasure and security on a newborn infant's face when the LeBoyer warm bath technique is used immediately after birth? Dr. LeBoyer insists that if his postnatal system of quiet, low light and a warm bath were universally practiced, most of us would grow up happier.

Rich or poor, illiterate or scholar, most of us have an inborn instinct about the use of water in times of stress. An eight-year-old, a battered child, recently confided to a friend of mine that he often took warm baths to relax himself. Once, feeling bereft because his mother had shaved his head as a punishment, he sat in a warm bath for four hours to overcome his seething anger and abject helplessness. He somehow knew that there was sedation and comfort in that warm bath, just as others instinctively know there is stimulus in a short cold shower. Although our feelings about water are to a great extent learned, they may also be part of our collective unconscious, for even the most primitive people used water in a variety of healing ways.

HOW WATER WORKS IN YOUR BODY

Water therapy techniques may be likened to the complex activities in the control tower of a busy airport, where takeoffs and landings are part of a total system whose components must all work together. Some planes land in a center runway. Some are directed to peripheral outlying runways, and still others circle the field, or in bad weather are diverted to other airports. Water can be used in a similar way. It can work directly on the whole body, or it can act on one area to create depletion or congestion.

An example of a direct application of water occurs when you immerse your body in a bath. In this case, the water causes the entire body to feel tonified or sedated. An example of an indirect application of water is the use of a hot footbath, or a cold, double wet stocking, to decongest the head or chest during a cold. Another example of an indirect application is the use of a shoulder shower, or an ice bag placed between the thighs to reduce pelvic congestion.

Learning the many techniques of water therapy is somewhat like studying the superimposed illustrations of the human body that can be found in the World Book Encyclopedia. You can view one segment, several superimposed segments, or the total picture, as each celluloid overlay details the circulatory system, the lymphatic system, the endocrine glands, the digestive system, and so on, until the final picture shows the body as we know it.

Water therapy looks simple and it is often simple to do, but most of its action is invisible. Water can work in either a simple and direct, or a complex and indirect fashion, and its special therapeutic ability can be employed in its liquid, gas, or solid state.

One of the reasons water is so effective in natural healing is that it stimulates the body by producing an action, which in turn produces a reaction. An example of this is the effect of ice after an injury. The numbing effect of the ice—the action—not only acts as an anesthetic and thus reduces pain, but also reduces fluid movement and buildup—the reaction—and this controls bleeding.

The Reflex Arcs

In 1880, Dr. William Winternitz of Austria discovered the startling fact that when water acts on the nerve points of the skin, the skin then delivers messages directly to a nearby organ, or indirectly through reflex "arcs."

These arcs connect the skin to muscles, glands, and organs. When water—either hot or cold—is applied to the skin, the reflex arcs stimulate nerve impulses that in turn travel to other parts of the body. This action is similar to the transfer of electricity that occurs when a light switch is turned on, or to the effect on a nerve when acupuncture is applied.

FORMS OF WATER

Because water is such a common substance, we tend to take it for granted, never realizing the great variety of its physical and chemical forms, which are as easily available to us as the flick of a faucet, making ice cubes, or boiling water in a pot.

Each of these distinctive physical forms of water—ice, water, and steam—must be used differently, for each has its own specific function in healing and in maintaining good health. Indeed, water's therapeutic action is so complex and varied that if water didn't exist, and someone were to invent it today, its inventor would become the most respected and renowned scientist on earth!

Depending on its form (liquid, solid, gas), temperature (cold, hot, ice, neutral), and pressure (light to jet), water will have a specific physical and chemical reaction in and on the body.

Cold Water

Cold water acts in several different ways. For example, a short cold-water application acts as a tonic, while an extended cold-water application acts as a depressant.

Basically, however, cold water is restorative, reenergizing, and helps build resistance to disease. Cold water can help reduce even the highest fever, relieve thirst, act as a stimulant, diuretic, and anesthetic, relieve pain, reduce constipation, and aid the elimination of toxins from the body.

Cold water is the surprising and needed ingredient in a series of excellent heating compresses (cold double compress and various cold double body packs). Unlike hot compresses, which get colder, cold compresses, when trapped by an outer layer of flannel or wool (or even plastic, for that matter), become hot from heat marshaled from within the body.

Ice

Ice, or ice water, is very helpful in reducing the pain of minor burns. Ice massage, or wrapped ice, is the preferred treatment for injuries, because the cold helps to control the bleeding and reduce subsequent swelling. This is the best of all treatments for all sorts of athletic injuries. Ice is an excellent anesthetic.

Warm (Neutral) Water

Warm water is sedating, relaxes the body, and when necessary it is an effective emetic.

Hot Water

Hot water (as well as cold) can be used internally and externally.

In an injury, heat increases blood flow and will act to increase any inflammation; as a result, hot water must be avoided in treating injuries.

However, heat can sedate, quiet, and soothe the body under many other conditions. A short hot-water application depresses and depletes body and muscle tone, making the body feel more relaxed. And while a long hot-water application both excites and depresses the body, the total effect is one of complete relaxation.

Some of the most important therapeutic uses of hot water are the hot bath to induce perspiration, hot compresses and foot and arm baths to reduce inflammation and pain, and contrasting hot and cold baths to quicken circulation and body reaction. A hot hand bath allays pain and spasm in the hands. A cold bath can be used when the body is overheated, or to control a nosebleed.

Steam

Steam is available by boiling water, using a vaporizer or humidifier; or utilizing either home or professional steamroom or sauna installations. Steam increases skin action and creates perspiration, which in turn cleanses the body from within. Steam facials open the pores and keep them clean, and can help prevent skin problems and acne. Hot steam from a vaporizer eases chest congestion. Cool moist air from home humidifiers adds moist air to dry winterized rooms, thus preventing nasal and sinus conditions, and eases a great many airborne allergy problems.

CLEAN WATER

Water has far-ranging and extensive benefits. Clean water is critical for all our metabolic functions, from respiration and digestion to the regulation of body temperature and the nourishment of body tissues. Water lubricates our joints and regulates our breathing. When we are dehydrated, we often suffer from a host of ailments without quite understanding why; increasing our intake of water restores and maintains our health and natural balance. Water is arguably nature's most precious resource and the single most important component for the continuation of all life on this planet.

Clean water is a necessity for a host of biological functions, and yet much of the water we drink ranges from the mildly polluted to the utterly toxic. Where does our water come from? Groundwater accounts for almost half of the water we use for drinking and domestic uses, such as cooking and bathing.

We extract approximately 40 trillion gallons of groundwater yearly. Groundwater is created when precipitation that has made its way through the soil becomes trapped at a subterranean layer of the earth's crust and fills in the spaces between the rocks. The places where we extract water, called aquifers, slowly fill up with water, which accumulates over thousands of years. Aquifers are also abiotic, meaning that they do not contain the bacteria necessary to break down pollutants that can seep into the water if it comes in contact with contaminants. The nineteenth and twentieth centuries have seen a massive industrial revolution that has also meant a vast increase in pollution from farming, mining, and industrial waste; as a result, groundwater is contaminated with pollutants that can remain in the water for centuries.

Tap Water

How clean is our tap water? Is it safe to drink? Potable water undergoes a number of treatments to ensure its safety for consumption. But some of the treatments the government uses to regulate our drinking water may be hazardous to our health. For instance, many scientists believe that aluminum used in treatment systems could be linked to Alzheimer's disease and senile dementia, while others have suggested that fluoride put into water to protect children's teeth may be linked to arthritis and even cancer.

Ordinary tap water usually does contain traces of aluminum. Because citric acid in orange juice has a potent ability to extract and absorb any aluminum traces, it is not advisable to use tap water to reconstitute orange juice concentrate. There is also a chemical problem if orange juice is used to wash down a buffered aspirin. The two substances bind to form aluminum citrate, which is very easily absorbed by the body.

If you're wondering why aluminum is a problem, we do know that in autopsy the brains of Alzheimer's disease patients have been found to contain a toxic mass of aluminum. A recent British study actually connected the amount of aluminum in local water supplies with the incidence of Alzheimer's in the population. Although it is true that the verdict isn't in yet on whether the disease is a result of exposure to the metal, it pays to be cautious about aluminum. It does no harm to be aware of possible sources of aluminum leaching: aluminum pots, baking soda, and some brands of antacids, which can contain up to two hundred times the amounts of aluminum we should consume in an average day.

Lead in tap water can also be a problem. Pipes in old houses and apartment dwellings often contain lead. Because the water stands all night in contact with the pipes, the first run of tap water in the morning can contain lead. There is a simple way to control this problem. In the morning, run the cold water in the bathroom and kitchen for a few minutes before use. Repeat this action any time the water has not been used for several hours. Running the water cleanses out water that has come in contact with lead.

If you think that there are lead or lead alloy pipes in your house, never make baby formula or a child's meal or drink with standing water. Always run it for a few minutes. Don't ever use hot tap water for drinking or preparing children's food. Hot water leaches out the lead faster than cold water.

Yet despite these scary-sounding implications, water treatment, including chlorine and fluoride, remains a necessary precaution against waterborne parasites and disease. Water treatment this past century has helped to eliminate, among other diseases, typhoid and cholera.

The Boom in Bottled Water: Is Store-Bought Better?

The bottled water industry has grown at twice to three times the rate of the rest of the beverage industry. People are paying hundreds of times what they pay for tap water under the assumption that bottled is better, safer, purer. But that is not always the case. While water companies advertise their sources—"spring," "glacier," "artesian"—to assure the consumer that their water is indeed pure, several tests conducted by the National Resources Defense Council (NRDC) have found that unsupervised bottling methods sometimes produced contaminated water.

New evidence from the NRDC discussed in their report "Bottled Water: Pure Drink or Pure Hype?" claims that bottled water marketing can be misleading or inaccurate. In the long run, bottled water need not be your only option. Tap water filtered with home water treatments can be as pure as bottled water.

Home Treatment Systems

As a consumer, you need to be aware of the options in home water treatment systems. The following treatment systems are some of the best currently available on the market.

Reverse-Osmosis Systems

There are many benefits to using a reverse-osmosis system, and a number of specialists agree that the RO system is the best currently available. The RO system requires either a thin film composite (TFC) membrane or a cellulose acetate (or cellulose triacetate) membrane (CA) to operate. CAs are cheaper as well as resistant to chlorine, but they do not purify the water as well as the TFC membrane, which removes approximately 90 to 98 percent of organic and inorganic chemicals, as well as biological contaminants, from the water. Although the RO system produces clean water at a very inexpensive cost, the system wastes water at a rate of 4 to 9 gallons for every gallon produced. A recent study also found that RO systems are breeding grounds for bacteria. Nevertheless, reverse-osmosis remains a water treatment of choice. Lono Kahuna Kupua A'O, in his book *Don't Drink the Water,* writes that an RO system for the home should include a KDF/granular-activated carbon prefilter. A dash of sea salt per gallon will return mineral balance and improve the water's taste.

KDF (Copper-Zinc) Systems

The KDF system was discovered in 1984 by the inventor Don Heskett. According to some experts this system, a high-purity alloy of copper and zinc, is the best system currently available. The KDF system is durable and low-energy, and it inhibits bacterial growth. The drawbacks of the KDF system is that is relatively expensive and cannot remove organic contaminants or fine particles. KDF is a wonderful system for use in tandem with carbon filters.

Glass or Ceramic Pitcher

For a convenient and cost-efficient water treatment, the NRDC suggests placing tap water in a glass or ceramic pitcher overnight in the refrigerator with the top loose. The chlorine in the tap water will dissipate overnight, and volatile disinfection by-products will evaporate. Overnight refrigeration also has the benefit of removing the unpleasant chlorine taste and smell from tap water.

Carbon Filters

Carbon filtration is an old method of water treatment in which water is literally filtered through a medium of carbon. Contaminants cling to the surface of the carbon and are removed from the water. Carbon is effective at removing volatile organic chemicals and certain types of organic compounds, but it is not effective at removing biological contaminants and many inorganic chemicals. The catalytic/adsorptive carbon filter is a good home treatment, but the filter cartridges need to be replaced frequently to prevent bacteria growth in the water. Carbon filters are most effective in tandem with another treatment method, preferably KDF, which eliminates many contaminants that the carbon cannot remove on its own.

Distillation

Distillation works by heating water to its boiling point, then sending the steam into another chamber where it is cooled back into water form. Effective distillation produces the purest drinking water available, but if a substance with a lower boiling point is in the water, it will recondense with the water during the cooling process. Distilled water needs to be preceded by carbon or KDF filtration in order to remove chemicals that have low boiling points.

Ozone

Ozone is a much stronger disinfectant than chlorine, but it has a half-life of only several minutes, so it cannot prevent contaminant regrowth. Ozone removes much of the unpleasant taste in water and has a clean, sweet smell. An ozone home treatment system should be combined with another type of water treatment to produce pure water.

WATER AND WEIGHT LOSS

It may seem counterintuitive, but if you want to flush excess water out of your system, you actually need to drink more, not less water. Water is vital not only as a temporary antidote to fluid retention, but also as an integral part of any comprehensive weight loss regimen.

The body will not function properly without enough water. Unfortunately, many of us have learned to ignore our thirst signals, and so we aren't aware of the amount of water our body needs. The result is dehydration, not only making weight loss more difficult, but also affecting the health of our bodies as a whole.

But how much is enough? That depends on size. Most of us have heard that we should be drinking about eight 8-ounce glasses, or 2 quarts of water, every day. For the overweight person, however, 2 quarts of water is not enough. The heavier person has a larger metabolic load, which means that his or her body requires more water to perform the same functions as a thinner person. As we'll see, increasing one's water intake rids the body of excess waste and actually helps the body metabolize stored fat. The heavier person is at a metabolic disadvantage and needs one additional glass for every 25 pounds of weight. The overweight person will need to drink more water just to keep the body as healthy as a thinner person.

Donald S. Robertson, M.D., in his book *The Snowbird Diet,* suggests following this schedule to utilize water most efficiently for weight loss:

- Morning: 1 quart consumed over a 30-minute period.
- Noon: 1 quart consumed over a 30-minute period.
- Evening: 1 quart consumed between five and six o'clock.

A friend of mine, a fifty-something businessman in the airplane industry, flies weekly for his job and spends half his time traveling. He is not an unhealthy eater, but his diet is erratic. He will go without food all day and then eat an enormous dinner before going to sleep. His exercise regimen is patchy at best. Athletic as a child and young adult, he was skinny up until 10 or so years ago, when his metabolism naturally slowed down as a result of age and his activity level dropped as job pressures increased. Several months ago, a colleague handed him Robertson's schedule for water intake. He followed Robertson's schedule without altering his diet or exercise regimen. I saw him recently and asked him what he had been doing—not only was his stomach and midriff trimmer than before, but his skin was clearer and his eyes were brighter. He looked younger and healthier than I had seen him in years.

As a country, we are becoming ever more concerned with our weight, and yet obesity levels continue to soar. We turn to quick fixes such as weight-loss drugs and extreme diets, which work temporarily, yet which ultimately are frustratingly unsuccessful. When Phen-Fen was introduced several years ago, this "magic pill" removed pound after pound off people who had struggled with their weight for years—until scientists discovered that the pill was causing heart murmurs and quickly plucked it from the market.

Water is nature's ideal "diet drug"—the more you take in, the better you feel. Reading the warning labels on some of our contemporary nostrums, I sometimes wonder if the side effects are worse than the medication's benefits. Water's side effects—better digestion, younger-looking skin, increased vigor—are hardly the kind you'll see on any warning label. Water helps the body to help itself lose weight—letting your body work at its optimal level:

- Water flushes out excess waste.
- Water helps to relieve constipation.
- Water keeps up the muscles' ability to contract, maintaining muscle tone.
- Water alleviates fluid retention.
- Water suppresses the appetite by filling up the stomach.
- Water helps the body metabolize stored fat.
- Water helps prevent skin from sagging after weight loss by filling out the cells.

Elsewhere in the book, I've discussed the pernicious effects of dehydration as a potential factor in ailments such as arthritis, asthma, and ulcers. The message is the same if you want to lose weight: A dehydrated body cannot perform effectively or efficiently, making it much more difficult to function, much less to lose weight.

The Colon: The dehydrated body funnels water from the colon, resulting in constipation.

Hands, Legs, and Feet: The dehydrated body stores water outside the cells, resulting in fluid retention in the limbs.

The Kidneys and Liver: The dehydrated body's kidneys do not function as well as the well-hydrated body's. When the kidneys are not properly functioning, the liver takes over some of the functions that the kidneys can no longer accomplish. But the liver cannot effectively do the kidney's job and its own job simultaneously. The liver's basic function, to metabolize stored fat into usable energy, does not occur. Fat subsequently remains stored in the body.

Water might not only be the easiest, most natural, and most cost-efficient preventive medicine, but it is also vital for sustained and permanent weight loss. Water works systemically, allowing the entire body to function at its full potential. Not all panaceas need be exotic or unusual to be effective. Water is our testimonial.

Knowing the correct water treatment and knowing how to use it can save you needless pain and expense, and help you to take more active control of your health.

The preceding introduction to the basics of water therapy gives only a glimpse of the vast range of medical uses to which water can be put. In the following sections we will explore in much greater detail, and with step-by-step directions, more than five hundred ways that you can use water to improve your health and to maintain good health for you and your entire family.

part 2
Water Healing Techniques

MEDICAL USES OF WATER

*W*ater's three forms—liquid, steam, ice—can be used in a wide variety of temperatures and, especially in the case of showers or whirlpool, different pressures. Water can be used internally by drinking it, or by forcing streams of water into orifices, as in an enema, douche, bidet, or nose or ear bath. And water can be used externally in the form of full or partial baths; showers, even on minute spots of the body; single or double compresses, or various body compresses or packs; hot water bottles; frozen ice bandages, or wrapped ice; steam in several different ways; and various simultaneous or alternate combinations.

Because water can be used in so many ways, it has an astonishing variety of health uses:

- *As a restorative and tonic.* Water not only restores the body's normal circulation and temperature, but intelligent water treatment, especially with cold water, can also act to restore and increase muscle strength, and increase the body's resistance to disease. Cold water boosts vigor, adds energy and tone, and aids in digestion.

Techniques: Cold-water treading, whirlpool baths, cold sprays, alternate hot and cold contrast showers or compresses, salt rubs, apple cider vinegar baths, salt baths, partial packs.

- *For injuries.* The application of an ice pack will control the flow of blood and reduce tissue swelling in most injuries.
  Techniques: Ice bag, plus compression and elevation.

- *To relieve pain.* Even when drugs fail, an application of direct moist heat alleviates nervous irritability and reduces pain. Both hot and cold applications may be used to either reduce inflammation, act as a counterirritant, or divert blood to other areas.
  Techniques: Hot and cold compresses, ice bags, warm or hot baths, hot packs, enema, paraffin baths, whirlpool baths, hot and warm or alternate hot and cold showers. Do not use heat on a fresh injury: it increases blood flow and inflammation, and therefore tissue swelling.

- *For minor burns.* Water, particularly cold and ice water, has been rediscovered as a primary healing agent for minor burns, such as grease, candlewick, and hot glass burns.
  Techniques: Ice water immersion or saline water immersion.

- *To reduce fever.* Water is nature's best cooling agent. Unlike drugs, which usually only diminish internal heat, water both lowers the heat and removes it by conduction. In reducing fever, water is far more valuable than any medicine, and it is the treatment of choice for fever, sunstroke, and heatstroke. The Brand Cold Bath technique, or cold baths, should be reinvestigated as adjunct therapy for typhoid and typhus fever.
  Techniques: Short cold baths, prolonged tepid baths, dousings, sponging, cold mitten massage, high enema irrigation, damp sheet packs.

- *To induce perspiration.* The skin is the largest organ for elimination, and simple immersion in a long hot bath or a sauna or steam room visit can stimulate excretion of toxins from the body through the skin. Inducing perspiration is useful in treating acute diseases and many chronic health problems.

Techniques: Hot baths, Epsom salt or common salt baths, hot packs, dry blanket packs, hot herbal drinks.

- *As a diuretic.* The application of water can affect kidney action to increase urine production as high as 100 percent, and can also help maintain the normal pH balance of the urine.
Techniques: Ice water for drinking, diuretic herbal teas, hot moist compress applied to lower back, various cold sprays, alternate hot and cold sprays, cold trunk pack, sauna, full and partial blanket pack, and other perspiration-inducing therapies.

- *As an eliminative.* Water is a perfect eliminative agent. It can dissolve excrement as well as foreign elements in the blood through irrigations and through induced perspiration through the pores of the skin.
Techniques: Warm-water colon irrigation, genital irrigation, drinking water, kidney stimulation applications, vapor, sauna, or hot baths, damp sheet packs, dry blanket packs, hot moist packs.

- *As an antiseptic.* Boiling water can be used to cleanse food and clothing as protection against viral and bacterial diseases.
Techniques: Immersion in boiled and then cooled water, immersion in chamomile or calendula (pot marigold) steeped tea, cleansing with soap and water.

- *As a laxative.* Drinking water is generally necessary for proper elimination of waste materials, and can be used for specific laxative and purgative effects to flush material from the bowels.
Techniques: Two glasses of cold water on arising, enema.

- *As an emetic.* It sometimes is necessary to eject poisons (viral, food, etc.) from the digestive system.
Techniques: Drink copious amounts of warm water, salt water, or mustard water. No other vomiting agent is needed.

- *To raise body temperature.* Hot water transmits heat and warms the body.
Techniques: Hot full baths, hot-water bottle, hot footbath, salt blanket packs, cold friction massage.

- *As a stimulant.* Water applications can revitalize, awaken, or arouse parts of the entire body.
  Techniques: Hot or cold baths, sponging, damp sheet packs, enema or colon irrigation, whirlpool baths, salt rubs, salt baths, hot or cold showers, alternate hot and cold showers.

- *As an anesthetic.* Water can dull the sense of pain or sensation.
  Techniques: Ice to chill the tissues.

- *As a sedative.* Water is a very efficient, nontoxic calming substance. It soothes the body and promotes sleep.
  Techniques: Hot and warm baths to quiet and relax the entire body, salt baths, neutral showers to certain areas, damp sheet packs.

- *As an antispasmodic.* Water effectively reduces cramps and can help overcome both hysterical and infantile convulsions.
  Techniques: Chamomile enema, cold-water or hayflower-dipped shirt, hot compresses (depending on the problem), herbal teas, abdominal compress. Water therapy does not replace the need for immediate medical care in the case of convulsions.

- *To relieve thirst.* Drinking copious amounts of water assuages the thirst and restores the alkalinity of the blood.
  Techniques: Drinking pure (glass-bottled) water, distilled water with lemon juice, water plus fruit juice.

- *For buoyancy.* Bedridden patients will feel better and avoid bedsores when the body is buoyed by special "strip" water mattresses. In burn centers, badly burned patients are placed in tubs of sterile water so that nurses can gradually remove the burn scabs. Temporarily disabled or paralyzed accident victims and those with severe muscular and skeletal problems always feel better and move better when immersed in a pool of warm water. Often those who cannot walk at all may be able to move freely in water because of the buoyancy.
  Techniques: For bedsores: water mattresses and frequent sponging. For muscular or skeletal rehabilitation: Use the physiotherapy facilities in your local hospital, because electric equipment is necessary to deliver the patient on a stretcher into the pool.

- *For mechanical effects.* Different pressures of water can exert a powerful mechanical effect on the nerve and blood supply of the skin. *Techniques:* Friction rub with sponge or wet mitten, dousing, streams of hot or cold water directed at various parts of the body.

TYPES OF WATER APPLICATIONS FOR HEALTH PURPOSES

Water can be used in many different ways depending on the health need and condition of the patient, as well as the facilities available for therapy. Among the most effective techniques are direct localized applications, water streams, full or partial baths, sponging or other friction techniques, steam for cleansing and detoxifying, neutral washings, wet cloth wrappings, or cloths impregnated with various healing substances. A special water therapy technique devised in the early nineteenth century is a cold compress or pack with a dry outer wrapping, which creates internal heat.

Local Heat: Apply heat to specific area of the body such as joint, chest, throat, shoulders, spine. Use hot moist compress, hot water bottle.

Local Cold: Apply cold to a specific area of the body. Use cold compress, ice bag, ice pack, ice hat, frozen bandage.

Cold Compress That Heats the Body: A cold wet cloth covered with a dry cloth, or a water-resistant covering, will create internal heat and warm up the area from within. This is called the cold double compress. It can be applied to any area of the body or used as a complete body pack.

Tonic Friction: Water sponging and washing combined with some form of friction, from a hand to a rough washcloth, produces a tonic effect in the body. Use cold mitten massage, cold sponge rub, wet sheet rub.

Sponging: Use alcohol, water, or witch hazel applied to a sponge to wash the body.

Baths: Immerse the body in cold, hot, or tepid water. Use footbaths, sit (or sitz) baths, full baths, herb baths, or pharmaceutical baths. Any part of the body may be partially bathed, as in arm bath, eye bath, finger bath.

Pack: A pack is a larger form of the double compress, or may consist of a poultice of clay, flaxseed, or mustard. An example is the hot blanket pack, damp sheet pack, hot leg or hot hip pack, mustard pack, mud pack.

Showers: Several kinds of water streams can be directed against the body. Alternate streams can also be directed against the body, or large quantities of water can be poured from a height. Use dousing, jet, fan, or alternate hot and cold Scots shower.

Shampoo: Soap and water used together on one or all parts of the body create a shampoo. Use to cleanse hair, or after sauna or steam room.

Steam: A vaporizer can cleanse the upper respiratory system. A steam room or sauna increases body perspiration and releases many stored toxins. Cold steam, as from a humidifier, moistens dry rooms in winter and is important in preventing colds and sinus headaches.

EFFECTS OF COLD AND HEAT ON THE BODY

An application of either moist heat or cold produces a series of internal responses, two of the main ones being tonic and its reverse, atonic. When there is a tonic reaction, the body feels invigorated, muscles can be used to greater capacity, and the body responses include reddened skin, slowed pulse, increased arterial tension, expansion of internal blood vessels, raising of temperature, increased production of heat, increased skin action, and increased total breathing activity.

An atonic reaction means that there is a lessening of tone in the whole body or a specific area, a decrease of muscle ability, and a feeling of lassitude. Among the body responses are an increase in the pulse rate, a pale skin, lower temperature, less skin action, less production of air from the lungs, contraction of the blood vessels, and lessening of heat production.

On the whole, heat sedates, quiets, soothes the body and depresses internal activity. Cold acts to stimulate and invigorate the body.

Cold: Cold water depresses vital functions at first, but the body reacts with greatly heightened internal activity.

GENERAL EFFECTS OF WATER THERAPY ON THE BODY

To Help This Area	Use Water Therapy on Skin of This Area
Brain	Face, scalp, hands, back of neck
Pharynx and larynx	Neck
Nasal mucous membrane	Back of neck, hands
Lungs	Chest—front and sides, across shoulders
Heart	Nerves around the heart
Liver	Lower right chest
Spleen	Lower left chest
Kidneys	Lower third of breastbone (sternum), lower dorsal and lumbar spine
Stomach	Mid-dorsal spine
Intestines	Lower dorsal and lumbar spine, abdomen, especially umbilical region
Pelvic organs (ovaries, bladder, rectum)	Lower lumbar and sacral spine, shoulder, lower abdomen, groin, upper inner surfaces of thighs, from navel to breastbone (center)
Hands	Head (brain), mucous membrane
Feet and legs	Brain, lungs, pelvic organs
Lower abdomen, groin, and upper inner thigh	Pelvic organs
Uterus	Spine of lower back, lower abdomen, inner surface of thighs, breast, feet
Bladder	Inner surface of thighs, feet, lower abdomen

A short cold application is tonic. A long cold application is depressant.

Use ice to overcome initial bleeding in wounds or pain caused by spasms. Use ice for 20 minutes, then stop for several hours. See instructions for each specific problem.

Heat: The primary action of heat is excitation, but it then lessens the activity in the body.

A short hot application depresses and depletes the tone. This is an atonic reaction. A long hot application results in a combined depressant and excitant reaction.

Effect on Skin

Cold: A cold application at first produces less activity, but the reaction causes a secondary increase of skin activity and a lessening of sensitivity. This numbness is useful for injuries. Cold stops bleeding.

Heat: At first there is more activity with a heat application. But the reaction causes less skin activity and less sensitivity. Do not use heat in the initial stages of an injury because it increases tissue fluids and bleeding.

Effect on the Nerves

Cold: A cold application numbs and paralyzes initially, but the final reaction is tonic, and it results in a vigorous feeling.

Heat: An application of heat first excites the nerves, but the reaction creates a lessening of tone, and the result is depressant. This acts to soothe, quiet, and sedate spasms and generally relax the entire body. It creates lassitude.

Effect on the Heart

Cold: Cold causes blood vessels to contract. The heart first beats faster, then slows down. There is increased force in the heart action, as well as increased tone and activity. Cold compresses or ice bags to the pericardium, the heart area, keep the area stable during any heat application.

Heat: Heat causes blood vessels to contract and widen (dilate). The heart action slows down initially, then gets faster. There is less force and lowered tone. Although this is useful in some cases, it is generally not advisable to use intense heat because of its effect on the heart.

Effect on the Lungs

Cold: Cold slows and deepens respiration. There is an increase in the amount of air breathed in and out, and an increase in the oxygen (O_2) taken in and the carbon dioxide (CO_2) eliminated.

Heat: Heat increases the elimination of carbon dioxide and makes breathing easier, as does breathing in moist air in the form of steam. There is a decrease in the amount of air given off.

Effect on Metabolism

Cold: Cold increases the carbon dioxide, improving cell activity and oxidation. It increases the amount of urea excreted through the urine. This is especially true after cold half baths. Cold baths increase the acidity of urine, even the urine of alkaline vegetarian diets.

Heat: Heat decreases carbon dioxide, results in less acidic urine, and decreases the volume of the urine.

The application of heat over a large area diminishes the acidity of the urine, and it may become alkaline.

Effect on Muscles

Cold: A short cold application increases muscle ability and range. A long cold application lessens muscle capability and response.

Heat: A short hot application reduces muscle fatigue. A long hot application lessens ability and response.

Effect on Blood

Cold: Cold increases the blood count, particularly the leukocytes.

Heat: Heat decreases the number of leukocytes and red blood cells.

Effect on the Kidneys

Cold: Cold congests the area and excites the function.

Heat: Heat lessens activity and takes blood from the area.

Effect on the Stomach

Cold: Cold increases activity and increases the production of hydrochloric acid.

Heat: Heat lessens activity and lessens the production of hydrochloric acid.

Effect on Production of Heat

Cold: A short cold application increases heat production, while a prolonged cold application lessens heat production.

Heat: A short hot application decreases heat production; a prolonged hot application increases heat production.

ALTERNATE HOT AND COLD APPLICATIONS TO THE SAME AREA

Therapeutic Uses

- Acute infections of the hand, arm, or foot—avoid massage, friction, or percussion. This spreads the bacteria to other parts of the body.
- Convalescence—for local infections.
- Liver—chronic congestion.
- Pelvic area—chronic congestion as in the uterus, or after an infection.
- Menstrual period—when delayed or scanty.
- Muscles—when atrophied.
- Osteomyelitis—chronic.
- Ulcerated varicose veins.

SPECIAL REFLEX EFFECTS OF SHORT COLD-WATER APPLICATIONS

A short, very cold percussion shower directed at a reflex area causes active dilation of the blood vessels in the related viscera.

To Affect These Organs	Use These Short Cold Applications
Brain (mental activity)	Short splashes to stimulate the face and head; also cold compresses.
Lungs	Chest friction, as in cold rub, or douches increase respiration at first. Soon they result in deeper respiration with a somewhat slowed rate.
Heart rate and force	Cold shower over heart or slapping chest with cold towel increase both the heart rate and force. After the end of the application, the rate decreases while the force remains increased.
Uterus	Short cold shower to the back of hip area or feet causes contractions of the muscles.
Bladder, bowels, and uterus	Short applications to abdomen, hands, or feet causes contractions of the muscles.
Kidney secretion (increased)	Short cold douche or ice bag intermittently to the lower third of the breastbone (sternum) increases release of urine.
Liver	Very short cold shower on liver causes active dilation of its vessels and increases gastric secretion.
Gastrointestinal	Moderately prolonged cold application to the middle abdomen over the navel increases gastric secretion.

SPECIAL REFLEX EFFECTS OF PROLONGED COLD-WATER APPLICATIONS

A continuous local application of cold causes contraction of the muscles and decreases the vital activities of the surface, as well as the internal area connected by reflex.

To Affect These Organs	Use These Prolonged Cold Applications
Artery	Cold applied over the trunk of an artery causes contraction of the artery and its furthest branches, e.g., ice bags applied over the carotid arteries decrease the blood going to the brain and head.
Brain	Prolonged immersion of hands in cold water causes contraction. Long cold applications to the face, forehead, scalp, and back of the neck cause contraction of the blood vessels of the brain.
Nasal mucous membrane	Prolonged immersion of hands in cold water causes contraction of the vessels of the nasal mucous membranes. *Note:* Holding ice in your hand will overcome a nosebleed.
Thyroid	Ice bag over the thyroid decreases its vascularity and lessens its glandular activity.
Lungs	Long cold applications to the chest contract the vessels of the lungs, slow respiration, and increase its depth.
Stomach	Ice bag to the area between the navel and ribs causes contraction of the vessels of the stomach. This lessens gastric secretion while application continues.
Pelvis	Long cold applications to the pelvis, groin, or inner surface of the thighs contract the blood vessels of the pelvic organs.

continued on next page

To Affect These Organs	Use These Prolonged Cold Applications
Uterus	Long cold shallow sit bath causes firm contraction of the uterine muscle. A prolonged cold application to the back area between the hips (sacrum) dilates the blood vessels of the uterus; this increases menstrual flow and decreases pain.
Kidney	Ice bag on the lower third of the breastbone (sternum) or on the same area of the back creates contraction of blood vessels of the kidneys.
Throat	Ice bag to the side of the neck below the jaw contracts the blood vessels of the pharynx.

REFLEX EFFECTS OF PROLONGED HOT-WATER APPLICATIONS ON FUNCTIONS WITHIN THE BODY

A very prolonged hot application to the reflex area produces passive dilation of the blood vessels of the related organ.

Function	Application / Facilitation
Heart rate	Long hot applications to the pericardium (area around the heart) and to many other parts lower blood pressure.
Respiration and expectoration	Hot moist applications to the chest increase respiration and expectoration.
Gastric secretion (increased)	Long, moderately hot applications over the stomach after meals increase gastric secretion and hasten digestion.
Gastric secretion (decreased)	Before meals, long moderately hot applications over the stomach decrease secretion, due to ensuing atonic reaction.

continued on next page

REFLEX EFFECTS OF PROLONGED HOT-WATER APPLICATIONS *continued*

Function	Application/Facilitation
Peristalsis (lessened)	Prolonged hot applications to the abdomen decreases peristalsis, relieves pain of spasms.
Intestinal colic	Prolonged hot applications relieve pain due to muscle spasm.
Bladder, rectum, uterus (increased menstrual flow)	Prolonged hot applications to the pelvis, such as a hot moist compress, hot pack, or shallow sit bath, relax the muscles of these organs, dilate their blood vessels, and relieve spasms in these organs.
Kidney or gallbladder colic	Large hot applications to the trunk, such as a hot pack, relax the muscles of these organs and aid in relieving pain due to spasms.

Alternate hot and cold applications to the same area cause alternating constriction and dilation. This increases the number of white blood cells in a given part, and so makes this technique valuable in acute congestions and inflammation, particularly in hand and foot infections. The same technique is excellent for chronic congestion.

Types of Alternate Applications to the Same Area

- Moist hot compresses, with ice compresses
- Alternate hot and cold partial or full body packs
- Alternate hot and cold shallow sit bath
- Alternate hot and cold foot or leg bath
- Alternate hot and cold arm or hand bath
- Alternate hot and cold vaginal douche or rectal irrigation

Hot or Cold or Simultaneous Hot and Cold Applications to Different Areas

With the application of either all cold, all hot, or simultaneous hot and cold to different areas, you can cause a withdrawal of blood from one area (depletion). This causes shunting of the blood to another area.

When heat is used alone, always end the treatment with cold friction massage with a washcloth or rough mitten. This helps the area to maintain the reaction obtained.

DRINKING WATER

*D*rinking water is such a natural, necessary activity that we tend to forget its many health functions. Whenever you feel sick, it is a good idea to greatly increase the amount of water you are drinking. I know that when I feel sluggish or overtired I tend to crave large quantities of two of my favorite bottled waters, Evian and Mountain Valley Water. Both are pure, taste good, and have excellent mineral ingredients.

FILTERING WATER

The question of pure water is an urgent one throughout the world. I keep a carbon filter on my kitchen tap, and I feel that it does help to filter out some impurities, especially chlorine. If you intend to use such a filter, remember to change it often. Although these filters will take out some gross impurities, they cannot filter out carcinogens, and an alarmingly high percentage of local waters contain toxic and disease-producing chemicals.

BOTTLED WATER

Should you use bottled water? In some states, such as California, a large percentage of people buy their drinking water in the supermarket. But I have discovered that some bottled waters in America are only reconstituted, distilled, or deionized tap water. Also, water is often sold in plastic bottles, which sometimes leech their petrochemical base into the water. This defeats the purpose of buying bottled water. Glass bottles are a safer choice, but be careful choosing what brand of water you buy. Some of my favorites are Mountain Valley Water, Evian, and Perrier. Other good brands are San Pellegrino, Poland Spring, and Fiuggi.

ALLERGY TO WATER

Lately, physicians have noted that many people are becoming increasingly allergic to their local water. Most patients never realize that it is the water that is causing their mild bouts of depression, slight or major headaches, diarrhea, or even arthritis. Various allergists report that as many as 50 percent of their patients are sensitive to local water, and prescribe one of the eighteen or so international and local pure mountain or spring waters.

Perhaps, like Michelangelo, you will discover a bottled water that will help you overcome a specific health problem. In 1559, he drank the Italian water Fiuggi, and it helped him to overcome a kidney stone problem.

Some naturopaths prescribe demineralized, distilled water, which can be obtained by the gallon from drugstores. Because of its absence of minerals, such water is said to act like a cleansing magnet by attracting unnecessary minerals in the bloodstream. Distilled water is alleged to be helpful in treating arthritis as well as some other health problems. However, the absent minerals must be replaced through food intake or judiciously selected supplements.

DRINKING WATER AS THERAPY

Some of the many health problems that respond favorably to drinking water therapy include fever, diabetes, rheumatism, arthritis, constipation, common colds, gallstones, edema, smoking, alcohol drinking, drug intake, digestive problems, and athletic cramps. See also the individual listings of health problems in Part 3.

Fever: Drinking 2 to 3 pints of cold water (about 40°F) can reduce a high fever from ½ to 2 degrees in 10 minutes.

Cold water lowers body temperature, absorbs the heat of the fever, and dilutes the blood. It also helps the skin and kidneys to eliminate the very toxins that have caused the fever reaction. It increases evaporation of fluids, and this also reduces the fever.

Fever patients should drink from 6 to 8 quarts a day.

Diabetes: Diabetic patients should drink copious amounts (6 to 8 glasses a day) of pure water and fluids to remove, via the skin and kidneys, all the unoxidized sugar from the body.

Rheumatism and Arthritis: It is helpful for rheumatic and arthritic patients to drink large quantities of water in order to dissolve and eliminate uric acid and other waste materials and to stimulate skin and kidney function.

Constipation: Drink 2 glasses of cold water before breakfast to help overcome constipation.

Common Colds: Both folk wisdom and orthodox medical practice advise drinking "lots of fluids" before the onset of a cold and during such an attack. Drinking pure, room-temperature water and copious amounts of hot herbal teas will flush the system and help to restore normal functioning.

Gallstones: Drinking 8 to 12 glasses of water a day will greatly dilute the bile secretion and flush the liver.

Edema: When the tissues of the body—especially in the feet—are swollen, it is necessary to drink several quarts of pure water a day. But it is advisable to drink it only early in the morning and in the evening—not in the intervening hours. If additional water is necessary, drink it in ounce quantities only.

Smoking: Heavy smokers should drink copious amounts of water to eliminate the cigarette toxins from the body and to stimulate the liver in its detoxification activities.

Alcohol Drinking: Drink copious amounts of water to flush the alcohol from the system and to help the liver eliminate the foreign toxins deposited by the alcohol.

Prescription Drugs: It is helpful to drink copious amounts of water while on a regimen of prescription (or hard) drugs. This flushes the drug out of the system after it is "used" and helps the liver detoxify the substances.

Always take yogurt, or acidophilus tablets or liquid, when on a prescription drug. This restores the necessary intestinal flora, helps achieve more normal elimination, and may help to prevent a yeast infection following long-term drug use.

Digestive Problems: Drinking cold water acts as a tonic to the digestive system, but it is hot water that aids and relieves chronic gastritis, hyperpepsia, and colic.

FLUIDS AND THE ATHLETE

Professional athletes know that they must drink water consistently in order to perform well. That is why many athletes travel with cases of their favorite bottled water or have it sent on ahead to every training camp and game.

Drinking water has an important role in sports. In normal life, we must drink a certain amount of water simply to exist, but this amount must be greatly increased when we engage in sports, especially competitive sports. This is due to the 2 to 3 percent body water depletion of such activity, and also because internal water intake affects both calf cramps and the fatigue level of the body.

Sports physicians note that it takes about ten playing days in hot weather for the body to accommodate its salt-conserving capacity and therefore advise athletes to drink large quantities of water before playing and during every break. They also advise adding salt, either directly to the drinking water in the amount of one-half teaspoon to a quart, or by swallowing 2 or 3 salt tablets and flushing them down with large amounts of neutralizing water. Such salt replenishes the supply excreted through urine or sweat, and greatly lessens the possibility of heat prostration. A former professional baseball player, amateur boxer, and jujitsu teacher, Dr. Jose

Rodriguiz, feels that such salt and water intake also helps in the necessary production of adrenaline and sometimes "acts like magic" in sports.

Dr. Rodriguiz also notes that before-game abdominal jitters are often helped by drinking acid drinks such as tomato juice. Avoid taking antacids for such spasms, he urges, since such substances contribute to the perpetuation of the cramps.

In addition to salt-laced water or high-potassium drinks, such as organic vegetable soups, herb drinks are useful. Chamomile tea will also reduce stomach spasms and quiet the body; linden tea will quiet the nerves and help ensure restful sleep the night before a game; and peppermint tea is delicious, refreshing, and stimulating, and is easily prepared in large quantities and served cold before, during, and after games.

Cayenne pepper in very tiny doses will help to settle digestive rumblings and provide a small boost in energy. For digestive disturbances, add a few grains of powdered cayenne pepper to a hot herbal tea: chamomile, peppermint, or linden are excellent. For energy, add a tiny pinch or several grains per glass, or about one-quarter teaspoon to a quart of pure grape juice, and sip as needed.

DRINKING WATER FOR NEWBORNS

I have often been asked if newborn infants should be given purer water than adults. The answer is definitely yes. The newborn child is susceptible to dehydration and needs water that is almost mineral and sulphate free. Because infants are susceptible to gastrointestinal upsets, it is also very important to have a water source that has a low bacteria count and no toxic deposits. Certainly, in the first weeks, the infant needs help in getting the kidneys to function normally, and fresh, pure water is essential in activating kidneys, causing perspiration, and maintaining internal heat balance.

If you live in an area with a poor water supply or high mineral and high sulphate content, you should definitely use one of the better bottled waters. Evian bottled water, highly regarded by French parents and their physicians, is available throughout the United States.

As the baby grows, it should drink the same water that you drink, except in exceptional circumstances of illness or severe diarrhea (see page 286). In these cases, use bottled water.

ICE

Ice has a numbing effect, and therefore immediately reduces the discomfort of strains, sprains, contusions, hematomas, and even fractures. The cold also acts to control any internal hemorrhage by reducing the fluid buildup in the body tissues.

Ice also has a secondary use in later rehabilitation of injury and for chronic spastic conditions. Ice helps to increase the range of motion, stimulate the muscles, and decrease spasticity and pain. Physiotherapists use ice massage, ice bath, or indirect ice applications in such rehabilitation. This speeds the patient's early return to normal or athletic activity.

ACUTE INJURY

There is uniform agreement that heat must never be applied to any acute injury. Heat has the opposite effect of cold. It increases blood flow and the metabolic rate, and thus increases the inflammatory response and production of tissue fluid. These are negative responses in acute trauma.

Ice, on the other hand, decreases the amount of pressure in the capillary vessels and lowers the extent of the bleeding into the tissue spaces. Cold decreases the body temperature of a particular area. This slows the total metabolic process within the cells of that area, and consequently lessens the cells' need for oxygen and nutrients. This reduction in metabolism results in a reduction of the swelling.

Another important benefit of the periodic application of ice is the prevention of hematoma—a tumor or swelling that contains blood. This is often the result of severe body impact such as occurs in sports or in accidents. When ice is applied immediately following injury and continued as described (see the alphabetical list of health problems in Part 3), the probability of suffering pain and edema—the retention of fluids in tissues— also diminishes.

WRAPPED ICE BAGS

A wrapped ice bag is the most effective initial therapy for most injuries, especially sports injuries. An ice bag is a waterproof rubber container. It comes in different sizes and for different parts of the body, and is available at most drugstores. If you cannot obtain an ice bag, you can achieve somewhat the same effect by wrapping ice in a towel.

Most specialists prefer to use ice in an ice bag, which is lightly wrapped in a dry cloth and attached to the injury site with an elastic bandage to keep it slightly squeezed. This compression reinforces the physiological action of the cold application.

In order to avoid frostbite or freezing, place a layer of fabric between the skin and the ice bag (the wrapping on the ice bag will do). Then immobilize the injured part by bed rest or elevation. You can easily remember the three related injury procedures with the acronym ICE, which represents the words *Ice, Compression, Elevation.*

The total length of time for ice therapy varies by injury, severity, and possibility of recurrent hemorrhage. Most professionals use ice bags plus compression in 20- to 30-minute sessions, usually two times a day. (In my experience cold is most effective in 20 minute segments.) But sometimes shorter applications are desired, up to four times a day. Most injuries respond within 24 to 48 hours, but some require up to 72 hours of periodic ice attention. Specific details as described by some noted team physicians, coaches, and trainers are given in Part 3.

ICE BAG

Therapeutic Uses

- Stop bleeding
- Relieve joint pain
- Relieve pain after injury
- Reduce head congestion (apply to head)
- Numb an area
- Check congestion
- Protect heart during heat application on other parts of the body or for heart problems
- Prevent swelling of sprain or contusion
- Check inflammation

An ice bag is a soft leakproof rubber container holding ice. It is one of the most useful and versatile of water therapies. It is also one of the several possible cold applications to the head—the others being ice turbans and "hats," ice packs, cold compresses, and sponging with ice water. Always start these applications with tepid water. (See further details on cold applications to the head on page 44.)

To fill an ice bag, first get rid of the sharp edges of the ice, or crush the ice slightly. For a head or chest application, fill the bag half full. If the back of the neck or the head is to rest on the bag, fill the bag completely. In either case, expel the air before screwing on the lid. Make sure to fasten the lid very tight. Dry the bag (a wet bag can freeze the skin) and cover it with a thin kitchen or hand towel. The covering is important because it makes the initial reaction less intense, and also prevents the body from heating up the bag (the reverse of what you want to accomplish). For this reason, it is important to replace the ice as soon as it melts because then it changes into a warm compress.

Do not apply cold continuously, but rather periodically. Also, rub the body part briskly with the hand between applications of ice.

ICE PACK

Therapeutic Uses

- When ice bag is not available
- When ice application is needed for large body area

- As a cold application around the entire neck
- As a turban for the top of the head
- When packing a joint to reduce pain or avoid swelling from an injury

To make an ice pack, empty about three freezer trays, crush the ice, and place it in the center of a large, folded bath towel. Fold the towel over the ice and apply it as an ice collar around the neck, or around a joint, or as a large ice application to other parts of the body. Use an intervening layer of fabric to protect the skin. Massage the skin frequently to prevent freezing of the tissues.

ICE TURBAN

Make an ice turban by soaking a large, light towel in ice water and winding it around the head. Place crushed ice in another small, porous towel and apply over the turban to the top of the head. Ice packs and ice turbans have the same action as an ice bag, which holds ice in a rubber container.

COLD APPLICATION TO HEAD

Therapeutic Uses

- Eliminate fatigue of the body or mind
- Prevent or control headaches
- Control faintness
- Use with other applications to treat loss of memory, worry, depression
- As cold compress during hot footbath, or any hot moist heat application to the rest of the body
- During attempts to induce perspiration

Bags, towels, and cloths can be used as various kinds of cold head applications, including ice "hats," ice packs, ice bags, and cold compresses. Short applications are very tonic and excite mental activity, as well as helping to decongest the head. Long applications of cold to the head will lower the temperature of the brain and lessen internal vital activity as well as the production of heat.

When cold compresses, packs, or turbans are used during perspiration-producing therapy, renew the compresses every few minutes, otherwise they become warm compresses. Also, stabilize the procedure by increasing the intake of drinking water. This replaces the fluid lost with excretion of toxins.

FROZEN BANDAGE

Therapeutic Uses

- Minor sprains
- Spasms that don't react well to heat
- Minor athletic injuries
- Some sciatic tension

I use these homemade frozen bandages for minor sprains, minor first aid, and the release of such spasms as do not respond to moist heat.

I always keep several of these handy ice aids in my freezer, because sometimes the body takes more kindly to these bandages than to ice. They are invaluable when you need to marshal internal heat within the body. Unlike ice bags, which stay continuously cold, frozen bandages gradually become warmer and warmer. Children love being treated with these special bandages.

Method

Plunge a dish towel in ice cold water. Wring out the water. Fold the towel lengthwise and in half. Insert it into a plastic bag. Place the bag in the freezer on a piece of cardboard so that the cloth will freeze flat.

To use, pull off the plastic and apply the frozen towel to the body. As internal heat rushes to the cold area, it will soften the stiff bandage. Soon the bandage will conform to the body area. For a sciatica attack that doesn't respond to moist heat, place an intervening cloth on the area and lie down on the frozen bandage. Often two consecutive bandages will eliminate the spasm.

COMPRESSES

Cold water, hot water, or liquified medications and herbs can be applied to any area of the body by means of folded cloths called compresses: cotton, linen, flannel, or gauze, in 3- to 4-inch folds. The thicker the folding, the longer lasting the compress. Because it is lightweight and easily available, a linen or cotton dish towel is usually my favorite choice for an instant compress, but sometimes larger cloths are needed.

THREE KINDS OF COMPRESSES

There are three kinds of compress applications.

1. *Hot:* Single or double. Sometimes called a fomentation (a relaxant).
2. *Cold:* Single inhibits circulation, flow, bleeding. Double stimulates circulation. This compress consists of one wet cloth completely covered by a dry cloth.
3. *Alternate hot and cold:* Sedates and then stimulates.

AREA COMPRESSES

Compresses are frequently named for the area they are to be applied to—for example, head, throat, joint, chest, trunk, foot, genital, or hemorrhoidal. Since many of these area compresses consist of large cloth wrappings, they can also be called packs. Most packs are actually double compresses.

The health problem that needs to be solved determines the compress temperature, duration, and whether or not herbs should be added to the water.

ADDING TO COMPRESS WATER

Apple cider vinegar can be added to either hot or cold compresses—except those applied near the eyes or genitals. When adding vinegar, use a tablespoon to half a cup in the compress water. For hot compresses, add the vinegar to the water being heated. Vinegar detoxifies and reduces inflammation. Witch hazel also reduces inflammation.

Other detoxifying substances that can be added to compresses are hayflower, oatstraw, and such healing substances as fenugreek, cooked carrots, oatmeal, raw or cooked onions, baked potatoes (all of which can be used as direct poultices on the area to be healed). Hayflower, oatstraw, and fenugreek can be used as teas into which the compress cloths are dipped.

A combination of mustard powder and flour plus water can be called a mustard compress, but it is most often called a mustard plaster (or pack). Mustard brings blood to the surface of the skin and is useful in overcongested areas, such as the chest in bronchitis; but it can reduce internal congestion elsewhere as well.

A few drops of tincture of arnica (arnica is an outstanding pain reliever for unbroken skin) can be added to the compress water while the cloth is being prepared to assuage the pain of strains or sprains. Use only on unbroken skin. Sometimes stimulating ointments may be applied directly to the skin (again where there are no open cuts or wounds), and the compress is then placed over the ointment. Arnica ointment, oil of eucalyptus ointment, wintergreen ointment, or the commercial Olbas ointment are useful for pain. Calendula (pot marigold) ointment can be applied directly to the skin under a compress in the case of sores, cuts, or prior bleeding.

HOT MOIST COMPRESS

Therapeutic Uses

- Relieve pain
- Stimulate perspiration
- Improve circulation of local area
- Relieve muscle spasms
- Help rheumatic complaints
- Reduce congestions of noninflammatory origin
- Relieve intercostal pain
- Stimulate the absorption of cellular debris during injury healing
- Relieve neuralgia

Always use a cold cloth compress on the head during a hot application. Hot, moist heat relaxes contractions.

Time Used

Long applications of 30 minutes to a maximum of 2 hours are sedative. They are thus useful for spine and sleep problems.

Short applications of 3 to 5 minutes are stimulating.

The effect of consecutive applications of hot moist cloths is similar to a vapor bath, paraffin bath (antipain), or an old-fashioned mud pack at a spa. As the hot moist cloths are replaced, that area of the body is alternately heated and cooled. This relieves the muscle spasm.

Sciatica, Internal Spasm, Colic

My father always said there was no better treatment for sciatica than a series of long hot compress applications, each followed by a short cold shower. Actually, all rheumatic problems, muscular pain, lumbago, and pain under and around the breast are helped by hot moist compresses. These applications can be repeated every evening until the problem disappears. In the case of gallstone colic or intestinal colic, or for relief of spasms or painful menstrual period, apply a trunk compress every half-hour.

Polio Breakthrough

Sister Kenny discovered the value of hot moist compresses during a 1920s polio epidemic in Australia. Desperate to relieve the pain of her patients, she remembered the water therapy her family had used when she was a child. She kept renewing the packs, which were left on for 12-hour periods. Most of her patients recovered the use of their limbs because she stretched and reeducated the muscles every hour after the heat application. These hot compresses prevented the muscles from shortening. (Water therapy does not replace the need for proper polio vaccination, however.)

Method

Boil water and have several cloths ready for immersion before each treatment. Use an electric hot tray to keep the water boiling, or else keep the previously prepared hot cloths covered in a blanket. You can carry several of them in a pail covered with a hot water bottle, a blanket, or newspapers.

Old wool is not irritating to the skin and provides the very best material for long-lasting hot moist compresses. However, large cloths of soft cotton or linen can be used.

Fold each cloth into three, and then refold into a narrow strip. Fold this strip in half so that you can hold the edges in one hand while you dip the center into boiling water. Twist tightly by the dry ends. Next, pull the ends apart. This helps to squeeze out the water. It is important not to use a dripping wet cloth! As soon as the cloth is squeezed out, place it in the dry cloth "carrier" and carry it to the patient. Several such cloths are needed.

If the skin is sensitive, stroke oil on it and stroke the area. Apply the hot cloth in a rocking manner, holding up one end and lowering the other. If it is still too hot, put your palm under the cloth and stroke the skin again. This relieves the heat impressions and partly cools the area at the same time. Do not lift the cloth up as this may chill the patient.

Cover the hot wet cloth with a dry towel.

Have the next hot moist compress ready before removing the first.

For very acute attacks of pain, as in muscle spasms, renew the hot compresses every few minutes. They can be renewed at 15-minute intervals, or as soon as needed, but on the whole, hot compresses can be left on from 30 minutes to 2 hours.

When there is a need for frequent hot moist applications to relieve pain or muscle spasm, purchase silica gel hydrocollator applications from the drugstore. They include instructions for use. There is also a wet-heat electric heating pad available from rehabilitation centers and some drugstores.

HOT MEDICATED COMPRESS

A hot medicated compress is sometimes called a stupe. An herb dissolved in hot boiling water or simmered and strained can be added to the hot water into which the cloth is being heated. A few drops of arnica tincture will help relieve pain. Homeopathic arnica tablets are also available for internal use and are exceptionally effective in relieving muscular and rheumatic pain. Gingerroot can be simmered in the water and then brought to a quick boil before the cloth is immersed, or ginger powder can be dissolved in the boiling water for pain relief.

Many famous spas in America such as the Golden Door envelop their guests in herb-dipped body wraps, actually the equivalent of large body compresses. These wraps, which usually include a small amount of wintergreen and eucalyptus and other herbs, can help to reduce pain and bring blood to the surface of the skin.

Another method of applying medication with moist heat is to apply pain-relieving ointments such as arnica, Olbas (a commercial product), wintergreen, or eucalyptus directly on the unbroken skin, and then cover the anointed area with a larger hot moist compress.

When it is desirable to bring blood to the surface, use a thin paste of mustard powder, flour, and water. (See "Mustard Pack or Plaster," page 125.)

Apple cider vinegar may be added to either hot or cold compress water.

COLD SINGLE COMPRESS

Therapeutic Uses

- Prevent headaches (use on head or neck)
- Reduce blood flow to local area
- Help prevent congestion of heart area (use on heart area)
- Relieve pain

- Prevent swelling from injury
- Anti-inflammatory
- Reduce temperature of body or part of body
- Relax during crying jag

A cold compress acts in an inhibitory fashion. The thicker the fabric, the longer the cold will last. The initial effect of the cold is contraction; then, as the internal reaction warms the area and the cloth, the flow of blood helps to break up deeper or nearby congestion, as in an injury or inflammation.

If there is a possibility of a neuralgic effect, apply a light cloth between the skin and compress.

Method

To make a single cold compress, fold a cloth (the size depends upon the need for which it is being used) in half or thirds. Dip it into either cold tap water or ice water. Wring it out thoroughly and apply. Renew cold compresses every few minutes to keep the cold constant.

To reduce even further the possibility of swelling, and to reduce the pain of a sprain or strain, you may add a tablespoon to a half-cup of either witch hazel or apple cider vinegar (no vinegar near the eyes, of course) to the compress water. Apple cider vinegar is also detoxifying. Hayflower water made with prepared extract, or from a handful of the flowers steeped in a quart of boiling water and strained, may be added to any compress to increase the detoxifying action and reduce swelling. Such hayflower compresses wrapped around the feet and legs will reduce swelling of the feet.

All three of these herbal substances act in an extraordinary fashion. Keep each on hand to experiment with. Witch hazel is sold in drugstores, apple cider vinegar is on the grocery shelves, hayflower bath extract is noted in the Resources.

Weleda sells Luvos Earth #2 for compresses, and Herbtrader.com sells French green clay on-line. These are used cold or hot in a cloth or applied directly on the skin. (See Resources.)

Where constant cold is needed for longer periods—as in sports injuries, abrasions, contusions, hematoma, sprains, strains, initial fracture (until professional help arrives)—use an ice bag, or crushed ice in a plastic bag. Keep a towel between the skin and ice, attach the bag with an elastic bandage to provide needed compression, and elevate the injury as described under each problem in Part 3.

Temperature of Compress

A temperature of 42°F to 60°F is considered very cold. Higher compress temperatures are needed for weak or frail patients: 70°F to 85°F. Compresses to the heart area should be about 60°F.

Usually, the colder the application, the briefer the application should be. See specific health listings in Part 3 for details.

Duration of Compress

Keep the compress on for 10 to 60 minutes. Renew every few minutes. Massage the skin under the compress every 15 minutes to help the body react properly to the cold.

Use up to two times a day, or more often when specified.

COLD DOUBLE COMPRESS

Therapeutic Uses

- Acute joint inflammations
- Hemorrhoids
- Chronic arthritis
- Gastrointestinal problems
- Pneumonia
- Sore throat
- Insomnia
- Congestive headache ⎤ Renew every few minutes.
- Hayfever ⎦
- Tonsillitis
- Ear infections
- Acute laryngitis
- Diphtheria
- Croup
- Measles

1. In early stage use single compress. Renew every 2 minutes to inhibit inflammation.
2. Follow by double (wet plus dry) stimulating compress to bring blood to area. Renew every 30 minutes or when dry.

The cold wet compress (a wet cloth covered with a piece of dry flannel or wool) is the invention of Preissnitz and is an extremely effective self-care tool. This compress has a general heating effect, as do all cold double compresses (abdominal, genital, throat, etc.). The double throat compress, the one you will probably use most often, is especially helpful in treating upper respiratory infections. Since these compresses are applied to one local area at a time, they improve the circulation in that area, increase elimination from that area, improve local nerve function, assist in the discharge of internal catarrh, and also work on the reflexes to the central nervous system of the part of the body to which they are applied.

COLD DOUBLE THROAT AND EAR COMPRESS

Therapeutic Uses

- Sore throat (neck compress)
- Earache (neck and ear compress)
- Tonsillitis (neck compress, neck and ear compress, or triangular compress)
- Mumps or swollen glands (neck compress or neck and ear compress)
- Bronchitis (triangular compress)
- Pneumonia (triangular compress)
- Influenza (triangular compress)
- Asthma (triangular compress)

This compress has a general heating effect. There are three different double compresses for the throat, neck, and ear region. Each is made in the same way, but is wound around the neck in a different direction.

Neck Only

This compress is used mainly for sore throats, and may be combined with the ear or triangular compress. This compress can also be used for tonsillitis, swollen glands, or mumps.

Method: Fold a cotton dish cloth or piece of a sheet in thirds. Dip it in cold water, or diluted or full-strength apple cider vinegar. Wring out. Wind once around the neck and fasten with a safety pin. (Optional: Wind a plastic bag over the wet cloth.) Over the wet cloth, or cloth and plastic, wind a large wool sock or wear a wool dickey. Make sure no air intrudes.

This is one of the most effective and important water therapies. It works as follows: The cold compress is "trapped" by the larger, warmer one, and the throat and neck are warmed internally. This provides warmth and increased circulation, which work together to help conquer the sore throat. It also works well on laryngitis.

Neck and Ears

This compress was invented by the renowned hydrotherapist Dr. Simon Baruch. It is excellent for mumps, swollen glands, and earaches.

Method: Follow the same procedure as for the neck compress. Wind the compress as above, but then wind again from the chin past the ears to the top of the head. Make a slit in this second compress for the ears. Tie or pin on top of the head.

Triangular (for Neck and Chest)

This is a neck compress plus a partial chest compress. It is useful in helping combat tonsillitis, bronchitis, pneumonia, influenza, and asthma.

Method: Apply the neck and partial chest compress as below. Then cover the wet compress with a larger dry kerchief or a wool dickey so that this second compress extends over the chest.

To sum up: These compresses may be used interchangeably, depending on the area that needs warming up. The important thing is that the first compress (winding) must be cold and wet. It may also be dipped in any of the herbal preparations mentioned for detoxification, especially apple cider vinegar. The outer cover must be wool to keep out the air. In an emergency, a second layer of brown paper (from a brown paper bag) or a large strip of plastic can be used underneath or instead of the wool outer layer.

A cold double throat compress will not only overcome laryngitis, but will help cure most sore throats. This technique is also effective in relieving earaches. I was traveling in England and Scotland recently, and not unexpectedly the weather was extremely rainy and chilly. I suddenly developed a slight earache which, to my later regret, I ignored. That night, however, the pain awakened me from a sound sleep.

Since I was traveling and didn't have compress materials, I was initially at a loss. Should I tear up a towel or a pillowcase, I wondered? I finally settled on tearing up my husband's white cotton undershirt. After wetting the strips with cold water—they proved to be limp but serviceable—I carefully wound them first around my neck, and then from the chin to the top of the head. I used a turtleneck sweater for a throat cover and wound a wool sock over both ears and a scarf over the sock to ensure an airtight fit. I looked like a Martian with mumps, but no matter, I slept soundly and awakened completely free of the earache. Despite continued inclement weather, that was the last of that ache.

COLD DOUBLE CHEST COMPRESS

Therapeutic Uses

- Bronchitis
- Influenza
- Pleurisy
- Asthma
- Pneumonia
- Emphysema

This compress has a general heating effect. A double, stimulating compress applied to the chest area or wound over the front and back is a most useful aid in overcoming breathing problems. This compress can ease a deep-seated cough and generally improve the circulation of the chest area.

Method

First Method of Application: Dip a flat cloth or medium-size bath towel into cold water. Wring it out so that it is slightly dripping. Apply to the chest. Cover with a larger dry towel. This loose arrangement gives immediate access to the chest. The wet cloth can be replaced by another cold one every few minutes, or cold water can be gently sprinkled on the bottom towel. This quick replacement is necessary to treat very acute upper respiratory attacks.

Second Method of Application: Apply a wet cold compress in the form of a criss-cross bandage over the chest and back. Cover the wet bandage with a large, form-fitting wool sweater. Lift off the sweater and sponge the wet bandage with cold water every 30 minutes. Alternate another dry sweater as a cover. When doing this, the patient must lift his or her hands and change position and sitting arrangements. This contributes to the healing process. Make sure that the patient does not become chilled.

Third Method of Application: Use two large towels. Dip each in cold water. Wring out. Place protective material on bed. Apply half of one towel to the back, half of the other towel to the back. Fold each towel over the chest area. Cover with large dry towels.

COLD SINGLE TRUNK COMPRESS

Therapeutic Uses

- High fever
- Hemorrhages: liver, pancreas, spleen, stomach, intestines
- Preliminary treatment

It is sometimes urgent to inhibit certain actions within the body, such as a high fever or internal bleeding. A cold single trunk compress can be used in these cases. Water therapy does not replace the need for immediate medical care in the case of internal bleeding.

Method

A cold single compress can be made from a large double- or triple-folded towel or from a folded cotton sheet. Dip the towel or sheet in cold water, wring it out, and apply it to the area between the shoulders and the navel. Cover the patient with a light blanket or large dry sheet. Renew every half-hour.

See also the water therapy techniques for treating fever and hemorrhages in Part 3.

COLD DOUBLE TRUNK COMPRESS

Therapeutic Uses

- Chronic pelvic problems
- Nervous irritability
- Chronic abdominal problems
- Insomnia

Method

Fold a large towel in half, dip it in cold water, wring it out, and apply it to the trunk of the body. Cover the wet compress with a larger dry towel or wool cloth. Cover the patient with a blanket or sheet. Have the patient rest for a half-hour. Gently friction-wash and dry the area, and keep the patient from becoming chilled.

COLD DOUBLE ABDOMINAL COMPRESS OR PACK

Therapeutic Uses

- Intestinal disorders
- Delay of menstrual period
- Constipation
- Chronic diarrhea
- Flatulence
- Uterine problems
- Weak nervous system
- Insomnia
- Sluggish liver

This compress has a general heating effect. Sometimes called "Neptune's Girdle," this pack technique is universally praised in hydrotherapy literature. It is very effective in toning the digestive organs, and also influences many distant organs. It thus acts as a general restorative aid for the body.

The way this application works on the body is so complex and interesting that it deserves special explanation. The combined wet and overlapping dry compress diverts a large amount of the blood to the skin of the trunk and the portal circulation section of the body. The portal system is capable of holding most of the blood of the body. Diverting the blood causes a contraction of the cerebral blood vessels and creates a tendency to fall asleep. This hypnotic effect takes place almost at once—unless a chill sets in, in which case it doesn't work at all.

Method

Use about 3 yards of light, coarse toweling. Wet half of the toweling with tepid water, wring it out until it stops dripping, and apply to the abdomen, placing one end at the side and bringing the rest across the front of the body so that two thicknesses of wet towel cover the abdomen. Wind the rest snugly around the body and fasten. For feeble patients, wet only that portion that touches the abdomen.

Cover the entire wet portion with a flannel cloth and fasten. Change the wet bandages every 30 minutes. Between applications, wash the abdomen with cool water and lightly friction-dry the area.

In acute cases, where a high fever is present, change the wet bandages every 30 minutes. Remove the compress when dry. Friction-sponge the abdomen and dry with light friction strokes.

In treating chronic digestive problems, the compress may be left on the entire night and removed the next morning. Cleanse the abdomen with cold water and friction-dry. This compress is also helpful in overcoming chronic insomnia cases.

In the past century, before the introduction of antibiotics, this water therapy was highly praised by physicians for its ability to help cure appendicitis and particularly typhoid fever.

Since the typhoid bacillus no longer responds to certain preferred antibiotics, this technique may be of great importance once again. It can also be used as a prophylactic measure to tone the body during typhoid epidemics.

COLD SINGLE JOINT COMPRESS

Therapeutic Uses

- Acute joint inflammation
- Ulceration
- Scalding

Method

Fold a cloth about the size of a dish towel several times. Dip it into cold water. Wring out the cloth so that it is wet but not dripping and lightly fasten it around the inflamed joint. Since the pain may be intense, do not disturb the compress, but lightly sprinkle cold water on the area every 15 minutes to keep the compress continuously cold. To treat burns or ulcerations, add vitamin E oil or ointment of the juice of the aloe plant after the acute attack is over, and apply the following cold double joint compress as secondary therapy.

COLD DOUBLE JOINT COMPRESS

Therapeutic Uses

- Chronic arthritis or nonacute attacks (wrist, hand, knee, ankle, foot)

This compress has a general heating effect.

Method

Dip a long, narrow compress cloth into cold water, wring it out so that it is wet but not dripping, and wind it spirally around the joint. Cover with warm flannel or old soft wool and fasten. Change every 30 minutes to 2 hours, or whenever the compress warms up and dries.

The joints may be medicated first with arnica lotion or ointment, Olbas oil or ointment, or oil of wintergreen to increase circulation or reduce pain.

HOT MOIST JOINT COMPRESS

Therapeutic Uses

- Rheumatic pains
- Chronic joint problems
- Contracting skin
- Gout

Method

Dip a cotton or linen compress that has been folded several times into boiling hot water. Squeeze out the water until it stops dripping and apply immediately to the area of joint pain. To relieve pain, this compress can be used on occasion, or several times a day, 6 hours apart. Wash area with tepid, then cool water, and friction-dry. The herbal ointments mentioned above for the cold double compress may also be used with the hot compress.

GENITAL OR HEMORRHOIDAL COMPRESS

Method

Use either hot or cold compresses. To overcome pain and sedate the area, use warm or hot moist applications. To reduce inflammation and tissue disruption, use cold applications. Both kinds of compresses work by acting on the local group of nerves feeding the sympathetic system of the area.

COLD DOUBLE GENITAL COMPRESS

Therapeutic Uses

- Rectal inflammations
- Inflammation of the scrotum or testes
- Inflammation of the anus
- Prolapse of the rectum

- Inflammation of the prostate
- Inflammatory hemorrhoids

This compress has a general heating effect.

Method

Attach a cold compress with a T-shaped bandage or sanitary pad belt and cover the wet compress with a dry flannel cloth. For acute attacks, change every 15 minutes until relief occurs.

For chronic rectal or genital lesions, renew the cold compress every hour, or when warm and dry. It may be left on overnight.

HOT MOIST RECTAL OR HEMORRHOIDAL COMPRESS

Therapeutic Uses

- Rectal straining during evacuation
- Spasms in certain hemorrhoidal conditions
- Straining of the bladder during urination
- Painful spasm of the vagina

Method

Fold a linen cloth the size of a dish towel into thirds. Dip it into hot water. Wring it out and attach it, using the same method as for the cold double compress. Renew every half-hour until spasms stop or area is sedated.

COLD SINGLE FOOT COMPRESS

Therapeutic Uses

- Pain relief

Method

Fold a large towel into thirds. Dip it into cold water and wring it out. Apply to area of pain, either folded on top or wound around the foot. Replace cloth often so that the area is constantly wet and cold.

COLD DOUBLE FOOT (WET SOCK) COMPRESS

Therapeutic Uses

- Overcome and draw heat from another part of body
- Overcome exhaustion
- Decongest head passages during bad cold
- Relax entire body
- Decongest lungs, chest, and bowels

Foot compresses are a very effective old country remedy. They were my grandmother's favorite way of overcoming the discomfort of a bad cold. The compress takes only an hour or two to be effective, but it can be left on all night. As it unclogs the closed nasal passages, the patient relaxes into a quiet sleep. This compress has a general heating effect.

Method

Dip long strips of cloth into cold water or apple cider vinegar diluted with up to 50 percent water. Wring out the cloths so they are wet but not dripping and wrap them in spiral fashion on the feet and legs. Wrap dry bandages over the wet compress.

An easier method is to dip long cotton knee socks in cold water or vinegar-water, wring them out, and pull them up over each leg to the knee. Pull long dry wool socks over the wet ones. Cover the feet with an additional blanket. After the initial chill, the area will warm as the blood congesting other areas (i.e., head, chest, abdomen) rushes to the cold expanse at the lower part of the body.

HOT SINGLE FOOT (WET SOCK) COMPRESS

Therapeutic Uses

- Spasms of the foot
- Excessive callus
- Neuralgia

Method

Pat the feet with light cream or Vaseline. Dip long cotton knee socks into very hot water. Wear rubber gloves to wring out the socks and immediately apply to each foot. Change every 2 to 3 hours.

HOT WATER BOTTLE

Therapeutic Uses

- Create instant warmth and comfort
- Sedate and relax an area
- Intensify any other heat application
- Increase perspiration
- Relieve menstrual cramps
- Relieve sinus attacks
- Alleviate pain

In the old days, people used hot bricks and copper warming pans to transfer heat to the body. Nowadays we have flat, portable, and inexpensive rubber containers. Hot-water applications must sometimes be dry, yet have the penetrating quality of moist heat, and the hot water bottle meets this need. A hot water bottle will relax the body, reduce spasms and pain, and hasten the healing process by absorbing cellular debris. It is a versatile health tool that should be in every home.

A friend who is a writer tells me that he uses a hot water bottle over his forehead and over the bridge of his nose to relieve the pain of a severe sinus attack. A hot water bottle can be wrapped in a towel and applied to the abdomen of a colicky child. Or it can be used along with loud ticking clocks to relax puppies who are away from their mother for the first time. Hot water bottles can also be used to warm cold feet and to relieve severe menstrual cramps. Several hot water bottles can be used together to stimulate a sluggish heat reaction in a feeble, exhausted, or comatose patient.

Fill the rubber bottle three-quarters full with hot—never boiling—water and wrap it in a towel before applying to any area of the body. If you have sensitive skin, apply either a vegetable oil or easily absorbed cold cream before using the hot water bottle. Leave it on the affected area until relief occurs.

Hot water bottles should not be folded because they may crack.

Hot salt, hot cornmeal, or hot sand may be wrapped in a double pillowcase, or a loaf of bread may be decrusted and heated if hot-water containers are not available.

BATHS

Many ancient cultures used baths for rituals and health. The custom of bath chambers may have been created by the Egyptians, and then improved upon and developed by other cultures living on or around the Aegean Sea. Bathing was also an integral ritual in Jewish tribal life. Even in the Dark Ages, when the Church frowned on bathing, the Jews maintained public bathhouses. This may be one reason this small group survived the decimation of the bubonic and other plagues.

The ancient Minoans left the remnants of bathing apartments in the palaces of Knossos and Tiryns, as did the very ancient Greeks who created luxurious bathing areas complete with heated water, cold showers, and plunging pools. We know from fragments of medical history that the eminent Greek physician Hippocrates advocated the use of baths as medicine. As one of the early and great clinical observers, he noted a direct correlation between the use of partial and full baths and healing of many diseases. Hippocrates was one of the first physicians to state that nature should be used to heal the body; he realized that the body's capacity for self-healing was so strong that nature needs only a boost to start the healing process.

My own favorite baths vary with mood and according to need. I like hot-water baths to relax and soothe the body and to overcome aches and pains. However, long hot baths deplete the energy and tone within the body. Cold water, on the other hand, restores body tone. In the case of pain, or when you want to relax before sleep, or if you wish to produce perspiration to eliminate toxins, bacteria, or disease from the body, warm or hot baths are effective. Otherwise, use either neutral, cool, or cold-water baths. For tonic effects there is nothing better than cold water. No matter what your own bathing preference is, remember to end each bath and shower session with cool or cold water.

To improve your energy level, vitality, and disease resistance, use the cold-water treading bath (page 86), or a version of that cold bath, every day.

FULL COLD BATH

Therapeutic Uses

- Stimulates the body
- Lowers extreme fever from disease or heat attack
- Acts as a tonic
- Promotes resistance to disease

Short Full Cold Bath: For Healthy Persons

A cold plunge into very cold water is an exhilarating experience. I had my first experience with the use of the cold plunge after a sauna in Stockholm. The first effect was a slight shock to the body, then complete pleasure.

Method: To duplicate the famous Swedish cold bath at home, first warm your body up with hot drinks (herbal teas are excellent), a hot steamy bath, or a hot steamy shower, and then immerse your body in a full tub of cold water from the tap. The first effect is chill, followed by comfort. A second chill will follow, however, so leave the bath very soon after you feel the comfort set in. Always end this bath with a vigorous towel rub.

Remain in the bath for 30 seconds to 2 to 3 minutes, depending on your tolerance. Many people who use this bath develop such a tolerance that they can remain several minutes longer.

This bath produces a sense of deepened vitality. All the famous American and European spas encourage clients to take this plunge after steam and/or sauna sessions, since the cold plunge completely revitalizes the body.

Do not use this bath if you have organic diseases, high blood pressure, nervous temperament, or if you are weak, very old, or very young, or have heart weakness, colitis, or hardening of the arteries. In these cases the body's reaction is usually negative.

The bath temperature should be below 65°F (18.3°C).

Prolonged Cold Full Bath: For Ill Persons

"Cold bathing is a power for good, before which all other measures must stand aside," said Dr. H. A. Hare of this antifever treatment, sometimes called the "Brand Bath."

Therapeutic Uses

- High fever
- Typhoid
- Typhus
- Heat prostration

Method: First warm the patient with a hot drink, hot shower, hot moist compresses, hot water bottle, or another warming method. Then gently splash the patient's face with cold water.

Carefully lower the patient into cool water, 65°F to 75°F (18.3°C to 29.9°C). With the hand, constantly massage the patient to keep the blood near the skin. Or wrap a damp cold sheet around the patient before he or she steps into the bath. Slap and rub the sheet constantly to create additional friction. The patient should remain in the bath only a few seconds. This is also called a wet sheet bath.

Dr. Brand's cold immersion bath was developed in 1861 during a typhus epidemic. Since then, the bath, combined with constant massage, has saved the lives of many typhus and typhoid victims.

This bath should only be used in dire emergencies, because it is a great shock to the body.

FULL HOT BATH

Therapeutic Uses

- Alleviate pain
- Eliminate fatigue after exercise (short)
- Reduce muscle spasms
- Relieve internal congestion
- Relax and calm the body
- Induce perspiration

Hot baths are useful to sedate and relax the body, to relieve pain, and to eliminate toxins from the body through the skin. They can also be used to warm the body for other cold-water therapies. I use hot baths (sometimes with herbs and medicinal substances added) after exercises or to help abort a cold. However, hot baths deplete energy. Make sure to apply a cold compress on the forehead to offset the rush of blood from the head (depletion).

Method

Fill the tub completely. Start running the bathwater at body temperature, or slightly higher, and gradually increase the water temperature until it is as hot as the body can tolerate comfortably.

Position the body so that the head is resting comfortably against a small rubber pillow or rolled towel and all parts of the body are completely submerged. Apply a cold compress to the head and keep it there for the duration of the bath. Remain in the bath for 2 to 20 minutes, depending on comfort and need. As the bathwater begins to cool, let a little out and replace it with hot water from the faucet. Do this as often as necessary to maintain the desired temperature.

If the bath is to induce perspiration, do not add cool water, but get out of the tub, wrap the body completely in towels to avoid being chilled, and immediately get into bed under blankets (or follow with the technique for "damp sheet compress" or hot blanket pack).

If the bath is not for the purpose of detoxification or inducing perspiration, end the bath by gradually letting out all the hot water and replacing it with cool water. As a final step, splash cold water all over the body. Get out of the bath and dry the body by rubbing it vigorously with a heavy towel.

Short Full Hot Bath

A 2-minute hot bath is similar to the cold application and helps when recovering from exhaustion after exercise. A short hot bath eliminates metabolic fatigue and stimulates nerve centers.

Prolonged Full Hot Bath

A longer hot bath, from 20 to 60 minutes in duration, is the water therapy for arthritis, gout, gall bladder, neuralgia, bronchitis, and the relief of muscular fatigue.

It is never to be used by very old, very young, weak, or anemic persons, or those with severe organic diseases or a tendency to hemorrhage.

TONIC FRICTION BATHS

The action of a cold-water massage with hands or friction materials such as sponges, hand mittens, or a loofah has a profound tonic effect on the body. Cold bathing plus friction stimulates and creates a circulatory and heat response within the body. All tonic friction techniques are invaluable for bedridden or weak patients.

There are four tonic friction baths: sponge bath, cold mitten massage bath, brush bath, and salt massage bath.

SPONGE BATH

Therapeutic Uses

- For weak patients
- For insomnia
- When body is overheated
- When water is needed for medicine
- To reduce fever

This is the simplest of the friction baths. It generally requires only several quarts of water. (In emergencies, as little as one pint of water can suffice.) Remember that a warm sponge bath sedates; a cold sponge bath stimulates.

Method

Splash the face with lukewarm water. Dip the sponge in water (or water to which a small amount of apple cider vinegar has been added) and sponge the body in sections, keeping each part of the body warm or covered. Salt or sodium bicarbonate can also be added to the water.

Rub the skin vigorously with the sponge until the skin is fairly red, moving from the upper part of the body to the lower. Be sure to rerub the upper part at intervals to prevent chilliness (especially when reducing a fever).

As soon as the sponging is finished, wind a clean sheet or large towel around the body and rub dry. Freshen the bedclothes, place a light blanket on the body, and take a restful nap.

COLD MITTEN MASSAGE BATH

Therapeutic Uses

- As a general tonic
- For people who get colds too often
- To rebuild body stamina
- For low blood pressure
- For bedridden patients
- For patients too weak to bathe
- To stimulate inactive circulation

This is a wonderful bath for bedridden or weak patients because the use of a coarse friction material plus cold water acts as a general tonic on the body. The consistent use of this simple "sectional" bath, with only one part of the body available for friction or air at a time, improves the blood's circulation. This, in turn, promotes the process of internal self-healing.

Method

Cover the body completely and only expose one small area at a time. Start the process by gently splashing the face with cold water. For exceptionally old or weak, or heart patients, it is also beneficial to apply a cold compress to the head and an ice bag on the heart area. This allows the circulation to remain within the other parts of the body.

You will need a pan of cold water, several towels, and two towel mittens, potholders, or hemp washcloths. Put on the mittens or hold a potholder in each hand, because the two simultaneous friction movements increase the tonic reaction. Dip each of the mittens in the pan of cold water. Start by stroking the right arm, rubbing and washing at the same time. As soon as you are finished rubbing, vigorously rub the area dry. Cover the area and expose the next area. The preferred sequence is left arm, right arm, chest and shoulders, middle section, left limb (lift the leg to get to back area), right limb. Next, turn the patient over, remove the back covering, wash and rub the back and the buttocks. Follow the same sequence of friction washing, drying, and covering. The patient will feel rested and reenergized and go to sleep more easily.

For detoxifying purposes or for help in lowering the temperature, add a half-cup of apple cider vinegar or several tablespoons of either coarse salt or sodium bicarbonate to the cold water.

BRUSH BATH

Therapeutic Uses

- To relieve asthma
- For weakened conditions
- As preparation for vigorous treatments
- To remove dead skin cells
- After a sauna

The best brush bath I have ever had was at the Studevant Bath in Stockholm. The brushing is routine after a sauna and cold plunge. It acts like a combination massage, deep pore body cleanser, and body tonic.

This bath may be used for invalids, or used by healthy people to remove dead skin cells.

Method

Soap the entire body with a nonabrasive, emollient soap or avocado oil. Dip a large non-nylon brush, hemp washcloth, or loofah into hot water and scrub the skin for 2 to 5 minutes in circular motions until the skin is red and the body feels invigorated. End the bath with a warm shower, gradually reducing the water temperature until it becomes cool.

SHALLOW BATH

Therapeutic Uses

- Note specific therapeutic uses under each temperature and bath duration

A shallow or sit (*sitz* is the German word often used to describe this technique) bath is a bath of 6 to 8 inches of water, up to the buttocks. A hip or half bath extends to the hips and partially up to the lower abdomen. These baths have a profound physiological effect on the body because the hot, cold, or tepid water acts only on a localized section of the body. A sitting or kneeling cold bath, used daily, will help build resistance and vigor, as will several of the cold footbaths.

One of the miracles of water therapy is its profound effect when directed to only one part of the body (see "Hand Baths" and "Footbaths"). A shallow bath that covers only the lower extremities in very cold, very hot, or moderate temperature water will alleviate a wide variety of symptoms.

Use a cold head compress for any hot application—this is necessary throughout the water therapy system. When possible, elevate the feet by placing them on a rubber pillow. When directed or if desired, this shallow bath may be taken simultaneously with a hot footbath or hot foot (or leg) wrappings.

A cold shallow bath of a few seconds will help to overcome fatigue and will invigorate the entire body.

Method

Immerse only the buttocks, upper thighs, and lower abdomen in the water. This is achieved by using either a hospital sitz bath (see Resources) or a bidet attachment, or by sitting in an ordinary bathtub in 6 to 8 inches of water with the legs elevated on a rubber pillow, or elevated and wrapped in hot towels, or covered with a blanket. Sometimes the feet are immersed simultaneously in a hot footbath. This speeds the body's response to the shallow bath.

During a shallow bath, keep the legs and the rest of the body warmed by massage. Prevent chill to the upper torso by either wearing a shirt or wrapping the shoulders and upper part of the body in large towels.

Use a cold compress on the head in all hot shallow baths.

COLD SHALLOW BATH

Before using any cold shallow bath, first splash face, neck, and hands with cold water.

SHORT COLD SHALLOW BATH

Therapeutic Uses

- Weakness
- Delayed period
- Inflammation
- Impotence
- Constipation
- Poor circulation in abdominal organs
- Vaginal discharges

A short cold shallow bath has a remarkable tonic effect on the body. This bath and the cool shallow bath may be used every day by normally healthy persons to increase abdominal tone. Because the bath promotes internal intestinal movement, it helps to overcome constipation.

For additional abdominal stimulation, rub the abdomen in an inverted U movement in clockwise fashion.

Water Temperature: 50°F to 70°F.
Duration: 2 seconds to 2 minutes.

SHORT COOL SHALLOW BATH

Therapeutic Uses

- Constipation
- Chronic prostate congestion

- Bedwetting
- Liver, spleen congestion
- Bladder weakness
- Hemorrhoids
- Chronic uterine infection

Add ascorbic acid to this bath to help overcome genital or bladder infection and promote hemorrhoid healing. Use 1 cup to 5 quarts of cool water and up to 1 cup of ascorbic acid (vitamin C) crystals.

Water Temperature: 70°F to 80°F.
Duration: 5 minutes.

PROLONGED COLD SHALLOW BATH

Therapeutic Uses

- Sedative
- Chronic diarrhea
- Inflamed prostate
- Severe hemorrhoids
- Dysentery

Unlike the short cold shallow bath (tonic), which promotes peristalsis and therefore helps to overcome constipation, a prolonged cold shallow bath (sedative) slows or inhibits peristalsis and will help to overcome severe diarrhea.

Water Temperature: 70°F.
Duration: 10 minutes.

TEPID SHALLOW BATH

SHORT TEPID SHALLOW BATH

Therapeutic Uses

- Quickly lower fever

Water Temperature: 85°F to 90°F.
Duration: 15 minutes

PROLONGED TEPID SHALLOW BATH

Therapeutic Uses

- Sedative
- Overcome uterine spasms
- Overcome severe colic

Apply cold compress to the forehead. Start with a water temperature of about 85°F and gradually increase the temperature until it is as hot as you can comfortably tolerate.

PROLONGED HOT SHALLOW BATH

Therapeutic Uses

- Relieve painful periods
- Overcome delayed periods (from chill)
- Relax vaginal spasms
- Alleviate severe sciatica (half bath, up to waistline, may also be used)
- Relieve hemorrhoid pain
- Overcome spastic constipation
- Promote perspiration (half bath may also be used)
- Alleviate severe cystitis

A prolonged hot shallow bath acts quickly to alleviate pelvic area and acute abdominal pain.

During this hot bath, apply a cold compress to the forehead and drink liquids freely. Begin this series of baths with water at body temperature or slightly higher (92°F to 98°F+), and gradually over the course of days and weeks develop a tolerance to 120°F. Prevent chilling, keep the upper torso completely covered, and conclude the bath with a warm-water sponging or shower in which the water used becomes cooler and cooler.

Water temperature in the bath can be increased gradually by removing 1 cup of water and replacing it every 2 minutes with extremely hot water. Each replacement will increase the temperature 1°F.

ALTERNATE HOT AND COLD SHALLOW BATH

Therapeutic Uses

- Abdominal congestion
- Prostate inflammation
- Hemorrhoids
- Sexual weakness

The alternate hot and cold water produces alternate sedative and reenergizing responses in the body. The general effect is tonic.

Method

Use two separate containers, one with very hot water, the other with cold water. First sit in the hot container for 3 minutes, then in the cold container for 1 minute. If it is impossible to use two containers, use the same sequence and splash water on the lower extremities. Alternate the hot and cold half a dozen times. Always end with cold water.

For hemorrhoid healing, add several tablespoons of ascorbic acid crystals to each container of water.

WHIRLPOOL

Therapeutic Uses

- Relieve pain
- Remove embedded dirt and dead skin cells
- Relax spasms
- Soften scar tissue
- Reduce inflammation
- Relieve pain after injury
- Reduce tissue swelling (edema)
- Soften adhesions

- Relieve arthritis pain
- Increase circulation of the limbs
- Relieve tennis elbow
- Relieve knee joint problems
- Increase circulation within the body
- Alleviate Raynaud's syndrome
- Help paraplegic and polio victims

Over the centuries, various cultures have discovered that there seems to be an extra healing force in natural swirling waters. Now, with the miracle of electrical technology we can purchase effective and safe portable whirlpool machines for the bath. We can also duplicate the technique of world-famous spas just by adding minerals, herbs, or salts to the water.

There are several whirlpools available commercially, but the most effective and reliable whirlpools are manufactured by Jacuzzi.

One of the outstanding therapeutic uses of the whirlpool is to relieve muscle soreness and fatigue. This is the reason many athletes and dancers purchase portable whirlpools for their bath, or go swimming in a pool with such whirlpool action.

Partial whirlpool therapy is often used by athletic trainers and sports physicians when an athlete incurs a soft tissue injury. First, ice packs are applied to reduce tissue swelling and loss of blood into the tissues and to reduce the flow of blood. The whirlpool is secondary therapy. When possible, the area is isolated so that the whirlpool is directed to the area that needs attention. This usually speeds tissue healing.

The moving water produced by a whirlpool can relax and at the same time energize the body. Also, because the temperature of the rotating water can be either lukewarm or very high, whirlpool baths are helpful in antipain therapy. Start the whirlpool bath at a neutral temperature and raise it to the tolerance of the patient. A whirlpool bath can vary from 15 to 45 minutes in duration, depending on the purpose for which it is being used. If you are following the whirlpool with a massage, wrap the entire body so that it stays completely warm.

Whirlpool therapy can help with circulation problems. It is a well-known aid in relieving chronic pain and the phantom pain that occurs after amputations. Whirlpool therapy will help to relieve muscle soreness and body fatigue, especially after vigorous athletic activity. It will also help to heal skin sores and infected wounds, reduce the swelling of chronic edema (tissue swelling), help reduce the pain of minor frostbite, ease scar tissue from burns, and help with weak and painful feet. Many physiotherapists prepare their patients for therapy-massage by first giving them a stimulating and relaxing whirlpool bath.

You can also use whirlpool therapy for Raynaud's syndrome, tennis elbow, knee joint problems, for the swollen joints of arthritis, and to improve the circulation of paraplegic and polio victims.

Do not use the whirlpool if you are sensitive to very hot water. This includes all persons with diabetes, varicose veins, advanced arteriosclerosis, or any advanced vascular limb problem.

EYE BATH

Therapeutic Uses

- Reduce inflammation
- Strengthen the eye
- Relieve sties
- Remove foreign objects from eye
- Reduce pain on or around eye

The eye is very responsive to water therapy. This is partially because the eye is so sensitive, but also because the nerve endings and muscles of the eye can be stimulated directly by water.

Method

Use a sterile whiskey shot glass or professional eye cup (available at drugstores). Fill it with tepid water. Apply directly to the open eye and rinse thoroughly.

To strengthen and tone the eye, splash cold water on either the open or closed eye first thing in the morning and last thing at night.

Cold, hot, and medicated compresses will relieve eye inflammation, sties, and pain that generates from the eye area. See the listings in Part 3 for specific instructions.

EAR BATH

Therapeutic Uses

- Remove hardened ear wax
- Reduce inflammation and abscess
- Remove foreign objects and insects

Carefully wash the ear out with a children's syringe. Use tepid to warm water.

HEAD BATH

Therapeutic Uses

- Sunstroke
- Head congestion
- Hysteria
- Some cases of epilepsy

Kinds of Head Baths

On Stomach: Place a tub or wide pot on the floor beside a bed. Lie on the bed with the face down and the head extended over the tub. Have tepid water poured on the back of the head from as great a height as possible. Continue until relief occurs.

On Back: Lie on your back with the back of the head resting in a shallow basin of cool water. Have a helper bathe the forehead, face, and temples. Continue this gentle application until the excessive heat is removed or lowered in the body. You may also apply a large folded cold compress to the head and apply the cold water to the compress. This will both intensify the action and keep the area colder.

NOSE BATH

Therapeutic Uses

- Acute or chronic catarrh

Although nose irrigation doesn't seem natural or easy, it is practiced with great success by those who wish to keep their noses free of pollutants and natural discharges.

Method

Add a pinch of salt to a half-cup of tepid water. Put the water in the palm of your hand and sniff it up each nostril. This is an effective antiseptic action.

A more professional nose irrigation spray that attaches to a Water Pik may be obtained for home use. (See Resources.)

DROP-OF-WATER BATH

Therapeutic Uses

- Inflammation
- Wounds
- Sprains
- Bruises

The capillary action of cotton yarn dipped into water can be used for the slow watering of plants. This same ingenious arrangement can be used to cool a wound, bruise, sprain, or inflammation when the cooling effect is needed for a long time, particularly when one cannot use ice.

Method

Place a pot with cold water on a bureau or shelf several feet above you. Situate it so that the injured part of the body is directly below the pot. Put one end of a skein of cotton yarn in the pot and allow the other end to fall over the edge and hang below it. The water will be drawn up into the yarn by capillary action and drop off at the lower end drop by drop.

PARAFFIN BATH

Therapeutic Uses

- Arthritis

- Local swelling
- Strains
- Gout
- Painful feet
- Bruises (unbroken skin)
- Sciatica
- Bursitis
- Tennis elbow
- Old sprains
- Stiff joints

A paraffin "glove" is an effective method of delivering high consistent heat to a painful limb or joint. In this process the hand, foot, or joint is immersed in, or layered with, a combination of paraffin wax and mineral oil. The wax coating raises the internal temperature and relieves the intense pain while creating a long-lasting sensation of pleasant heat. This type of bath was invented in France in the early part of the twentieth century and is used in hospitals by physiotherapists and in many European spas that specialize in the treatment of arthritis. The bath can be created at home in a double boiler or with special equipment available from rehabilitation mail-order firms. (See Resources.)

The instructions for the ratio of paraffin to mineral oil are available from each manufacturer, but usually it takes an hour or more to melt the 2 to 4 pounds of paraffin wax and 4 tablespoons of mineral oil that are used.

Method

Melt the wax in a double boiler until there is a thin film on the top. Add the mineral oil. Meanwhile, carefully wash the area to be applied. Dip the area quickly into the wax. (If you are treating your hands, hold your fingers apart.) Remove the body part until the wax solidifies. Repeat the process until a thick wax glove is formed.

Wrap the affected part in plastic or in a towel. Leave the wax on for 15 to 40 minutes, and then peel it off. The paraffin can be stored and used again. After a paraffin bath the skin is extremely smooth, soft, moist, and supple, and it is much easier to massage.

At Maine Chance, a noted American spa, women are given total body paraffin treatments prior to certain massage therapies in order to completely relax the body.

If you use a thermometer, the temperature of the wax should vary between 126°F and 130°F. Do not use a paraffin bath if you have skin infections, peripheral vascular disease, or any condition of disturbed internal heat or intolerance to heat. Occasionally some persons react to this treatment with temporary dermatitis.

RUBBER HAND AND FOOTBATH

Therapeutic Uses

- Relieve pain of the hands or feet
- Overcome exceptional stiffness of the hands or feet

Anoint the hand or foot with a pain-relieving ointment such as arnica, Olbas, methyl salicylate, or menthol, and place it in a large rubber or surgical glove or a waterproof bag. Close or tape the glove or bag and plunge the hand or foot into extremely hot water (as hot as you can tolerate). The air layer and the rubber protection allow the limb to obtain a much hotter treatment than could normally be achieved, and this prepares stiff or painful parts for massage therapy. (See also "Paraffin Bath," page 82.)

This bath may be given every day if needed. The temperature may be as high as 120°F. The bath time varies between 10 and 30 minutes.

FOOTBATHS

The feet comprise 10 percent of the total body surface. Partial immersion of the feet up to the ankles or calves in hot, cold, or tepid water causes reflex contractions in many other parts of the body, including the liver, head, and pelvic organs. The body's reaction to a cold footbath is longer lasting than to a hot footbath.

Therapeutic Uses

- For reflex action on other organs
- To cause contractions in other organs
- To divert blood congestion from head, chest, or lower organs
- As a preliminary to other treatments
- As an adjunct to other treatments

See special details under each type of footbath. See also "Mustard Pack or Plaster" (page 125) or "Herb and Medicated Baths" (page 99).

SHORT COLD-WATER TREADING

Therapeutic Uses

- Weakness
- Insomnia
- Poor circulation
- Exhaustion
- Varicose veins
- Aching feet
- Habitual cold feet
- Catarrhal condition of nose, throat, bronchial tubes
- Weak ankles
- Chilblains
- Nervousness

I love cold-water treading because it produces a feeling of euphoria and good health. Cold-water treading, or a cold-water whirlpool footbath, reduces the feeling of heat in the summer and helps to reenergize the body. It is the most important of the preventive water treatments because it builds up resistance to disease and physical vigor within the body. It is no substitute for exercise, of course, but it should be a key part of body care.

Such footbaths help to overcome postexercise leg aches. My jogging friends now take a full warm-hot bath to relieve their muscles and add a nightly, before-bedtime walk in cold water. They report they no longer have any of the leg cramps that plague many runners.

Method

Fill the bathtub with cold water up to the ankles or, for a deeper effect, with enough water to cover the calves. Enter the tub and hold on to a stationary wall grip. March in place for 5 seconds to 5 minutes. In warm or hot weather, walk around barefoot afterward, or wipe the feet vigorously with a towel.

The same effect can also be achieved by sitting on the edge of a tub with a whirlpool motor making a swirling movement in the water, or by sitting and constantly moving the feet and rubbing the soles against a rough surface.

Children, invalids, and postoperative patients can duplicate this effect by sitting and splashing their feet in a large dishpan filled with cold water. Rub the soles of the feet along the bottom of the container for several seconds. Do not allow weakened or feeble persons to become chilled. The amount of time can be increased week by week.

Walking in wet grass is also strengthening.

Water Temperature: 50°F to 60°F.
Duration: Several seconds to 10 minutes. Do this twice a day, morning and late afternoon.

Warning: Treading is addictive!

Cold toe and footbaths should not be used if the following conditions exist: rheumatism of toes and ankles, sciatica, neuralgia of the bladder, pelvic inflammation, irritable bladder or rectum.

SHORT COLD SHALLOW TOE BATH

Therapeutic Uses

- Create intense reaction in pelvic area
- Decongest lungs
- Decongest head

Method

Add ice cubes to a small amount of cold water in the bathtub or in a large dishpan. Dip the toes for 30 seconds. Rub the entire foot vigorously. Return the toes to the bath and keep repeating the action until the feet become red. End the treatment by rubbing the feet dry. Rapidly tap the sole of the foot.

SHORT COLD RUNNING WATER FOOTBATH

Therapeutic Uses

- Insomnia
- General fatigue

- Congestion in head
- Moderate depression

Method

Sit on the edge of the bathtub. Place your feet and ankles under cold running tap water for several seconds to several minutes depending on your tolerance for cold.

PROLONGED COLD FOOTBATH

Therapeutic Uses

- Sprains
- Inflamed bunions

Method

First, warm the feet under pleasantly hot water. Run moderately cold water into the tub and soak the feet to just below the ankles, or if working on ankle sprain, above the ankles. (See also "Alternate Hot and Cold Footbath" for sprain.)

Water Temperature: 60°F to 70°F.
Duration: About 10 minutes.

Do not use during menstruation, bladder infection, or if there is any inflammation of the chest, abdomen, or pelvic organs.

SHORT WARM FOOTBATH

Therapeutic Uses

- When vigorous cold footbaths cannot be used
- For soreness of the neck
- For circulation problems
- As preparation for cold footbaths
- To overcome congestion in other parts of the body

The warm footbath is more comfortable for the very young, the very weak, and the very old. It should not be used by those whose feet perspire profusely.

Method

Run warm water from the tap into the tub and soak the feet for several minutes.

Water Temperature: 80°F to 92°F.

To achieve a temperature of 85°F, use 1 quart of boiling water to 4 quarts of cold water. To achieve a temperature of 92°F, use 1 quart of boiling water to 3 quarts of cold water.

HOT FOOTBATH

Therapeutic Uses

- Relieve cramps in feet and legs
- Overcome insomnia
- Relieve pain of gout
- Prepare body for any hot-water therapy
- Relieve menstrual cramps
- Relieve neuralgic pains
- Relieve sore throat or cold

Hot footbaths are an excellent water therapy for drawing blood from inflamed parts of the body, or drawing congestion away from an organ. Hot footbaths will speed up the body's reaction to a salt massage bath or a shallow (sit or hip) bath.

Method

Use a large dishpan or the bathtub. Start with warm water and increase the heat until it is as hot as you can tolerate. If you have no bath thermometer, use 1 quart of boiling water to 2 quarts of cold water to produce a hot bath at 106°F, or 2 quarts of boiling water and 4 quarts of cold water for a gallon and a half at 106°F. If the water gets cool, withdraw 1 cup of water and replace with 2 cups of boiling water.

Renew a cold compress to the forehead every few minutes to prevent head congestion.

End every hot treatment with a lukewarm, then cool sponging or shower directed to the soles of the feet. Wrap the feet in a towel and dry carefully. Keep them wrapped for about 15 minutes.

When the hot footbath is used to relieve a sore throat or to abort a cold, add 1 tablespoon mustard powder to 1 quart of hot water and add this mixture to the footbath.

When the hot footbath is used in preparation for perspiration-inducing water therapies, add hayflower extract or strong hayflower tea or oatstraw tea. Or add a tablespoon of a stimulating herb powder, such as mustard; $1/8$ teaspoon of powdered cayenne pepper; or $1/2$ teaspoon of powdered ginger or strong rosemary tea or rosemary extract. Dissolve any ingredient in hot water before adding it to the footbath. Use only hayflower or oatstraw if there are open sores or broken skin.

Water Temperature: 106°F to 115°F.
Duration: 10 to 30 minutes, depending on the case and tolerance to heat.

HOT AND COLD CONTRAST FOOTBATH

Hot Water: 100°F to 110°F   **Cold Water: 40°F to 55°F**

1. 3 minutes	2. 1 minute
3. 3 minutes	4. 1 minute
5. 3 minutes	6. 1 minute
7. 3 minutes	8. 1 minute
9. 3 minutes	

ALTERNATE HOT AND COLD FOOTBATH

Therapeutic Uses

- Toothache
- Headache (use cold compress on head)

- Neuralgia
- Passive swelling of the ankles
- Foot infections
- Chilblains
- Catarrh
- Blood poisoning
- Congestion of abdomen
- To warm up the body for other treatments
- In addition to some other water therapies
- Congestion of pelvic organs
- Cold body
- Cold feet

An alternate hot and cold footbath is a very useful water therapy because the heat sedates, and the cold stimulates the feet and other parts of the body connected by reflex to the feet. This alternate bath is frequently used in treating sprained ankles.

Method

Use two containers. Fill one with hot water (100°F to 110°F), the other with cold tap water (about 60°F). Steep both feet up to the ankles in the hot water for 3 minutes. Withdraw and plunge the feet into the container of cold water for 20 to 30 seconds. Repeat the process 3 times. End with cold water. Carefully wipe the feet dry.

The beneficial effect of this bath lasts quite a long time.

ALTERNATE HOT AND COLD LEG BATH

Therapeutic Uses

- Insomnia
- Pulmonary congestion
- Ovarian congestion
- Suppressed menstruation
- Painful period
- Pelvic pain

Method

Follow the same procedure as for the "Alternate Hot and Cold Footbath" on page 90, but plunge feet into the water up to the calves. Keep feet in the hot bath for 2 minutes; in the cold bath for 20 seconds. Repeat 6 times.

Do not use this bath if cystitis (bladder infection) or any congestion of the prostate, uterus, or kidney is present.

HAYFLOWER FOOTBATHS

Therapeutic Uses

- Heal open cuts on feet
- Reduce inflammation of nail bed on toe
- Control profuse sweating of feet
- Overcome discomfort of tight shoes
- Reduce hematoma (tissue filled with blood)

Hayflower footbaths are a wonderful remedy for certain foot problems, and they also can be used to induce detoxification in other areas of the body. (See "Baths" and "Hand Baths" sections.)

Method

Make a strong hayflower tea by pouring a quart of boiling water over 1 to 2 handfuls of dried hayflower blossoms. Steep for 15 to 25 minutes (the longer the better), strain, and when cold add to the footbath of your choice.

The temperature of most hayflower footbaths should be tepid (about 85°F). The baths may last from a few minutes to about 15 minutes or slightly longer, depending on comfort. End each hayflower footbath with a cold sponging and vigorous towel drying.

For swollen feet use a short cold footbath (a few minutes), or a swift cold jet shower to the feet, and then apply hayflower compresses. The herb helps the pores of the skin to open and thus encourages discharge of internally stored toxins.

Hayflower is available in extract form from Biokosma, a Swiss firm. It is distributed in the United States by Weleda. Dried hayflower is available from local or mail-order suppliers. (See Resources.)

OATSTRAW FOOTBATHS

Therapeutic Uses

- Sore feet
- Foot blisters
- Knots on feet
- Pain of chronic gout, arthritis, rheumatism
- Sores that develop pus
- Ingrown toenails

Method

Pour a handful or two of oatstraw (depending on strength of preparation desired) into a quart of boiling water and simmer for 20 to 30 minutes. Steep for 30 minutes or so, strain, and when cold add to a hot footbath to create a tepid footbath. Sponge feet with cold water and dry with a coarse towel.

Oatstraw is a very strong detoxifier. Repeat this procedure only 3 times a week, 15 minutes at a time, until the condition clears up. Repeat only twice a week for persons in a weakened condition.

HAND BATHS

*P*artial hand baths act directly on the hands and work by reflex action on other areas of the body. Like footbaths, they can have a profound effect in alleviating any number of ailments. See pages 29–30 for reflex areas.

COLD HAND BATHS

Therapeutic Uses

- Control excessive perspiration of hands
- Lower temperature during ear inflammation
- Check nosebleed
- Relieve sunstroke or overheating

Ice held in the hand or hands will check a nosebleed. To prevent future nosebleeds, frequently immerse hands in cold water of 45°F to 60°F, 3 to 5 minutes at a time. Dry hands with a coarse towel.

Excessive perspiration of the hands can also be controlled by frequent cold-water hand baths, as above.

Cold-water baths can be used both to lower the temperature of the external auditory ear canal, and to lessen the pressure of the arteries in the brain.

Whenever there is a wound or inflammation on the arms or hands, dip the hands up to the elbow in cold hayflower water. To do this, add a tablespoon of hayflower bath extract (Biokosma) to a quart of tepid water and let cool; alternatively, steep a handful of dried hayflower blossoms in a quart of boiling water for 20 to 30 minutes (the longer the better), then let the water cool. It is not necessary to strain out the flowers. Keep the hand or arm immersed in the bath for 15 minutes. Dry well afterward.

HOT HAND BATH

Therapeutic Uses

- Chronic skin diseases
- Local inflammations
- Writer's cramp
- Telegrapher's cramp
- Needleperson's cramp
- Asthma
- Emphysema
- In preparation for cold-water therapy such as cold half bath or cold shower
- Abscess of nail tip
- Inflammation of nail tip
- Tennis player's wrist

For most of the above problems, soak hands in hot water for several seconds to several minutes, depending on your tolerance. Repeat 3 to 4 times a day, or as often as needed. While your hands are soaking, move your fingers to increase circulation. Cool the hands briefly with a cold-water splash and dry carefully.

Chronic asthma attacks may be alleviated by plunging hands and forearms in very hot water for several seconds. Repeat 3 to 4 times a day. Follow each hot immersion with a brief cold splash or sponging and dry the hands.

An inflammation that occurs at the nail bed and causes pus is called a felon or whitlow. Felons are terribly painful. Both the inflammation and pain will be reduced by immersing the arm up to the elbow in hot water for 10 seconds several times a day. Hayflower extract or strong hayflower tea can be added to this water to increase the anti-inflammation effect.

ALTERNATE HOT AND COLD HAND BATH

Therapeutic Uses

- As general tonic to improve circulation of wrists and hands
- After treatment for fracture
- After treatment for wrist sprains
- To help control mild hemorrhages in other parts of the body
- To help relieve minor frostbite (chilblains)
- For cold hands

Prepare two containers: one with extremely hot water (as hot as you can tolerate) and one with very cold water.

Plunge hands in hot water for 3 minutes. Withdraw them and plunge them into cold water for half a minute. Repeat 3 times. Always end this alternate bath with cold water in order to restore muscle and internal tone.

For very cold hands, start with a cold-water rub, then alternate between the hot and cold immersions.

HERB AND MEDICATED BATHS

*M*any herb and pharmaceutical substances can be added to baths to produce special effects.

Water by itself has a remarkable, almost magic ability to alter the body state. Depending on the specific need, water will decrease or increase muscle tone, reduce pain, or generate energy. The addition of certain herbal and pharmaceutical substances to the water is a twin present to the body. Some herbs soothe, others sedate or stimulate, and others soften the skin. Most important is the ability of some substances to hasten perspiration, to stimulate release of stored toxins from within the body. This ability helps to overcome many acute attacks and can improve a chronic condition.

All of the following substances are excellent, and some have overlapping effects. I suggest you try each of them at various times in order to note your personal reaction. Then, if you need any of these substances in an emergency, you will know which work the most effectively for you.

Oatmeal: Excellent for skin problems.

Salt: Large amounts of salt added to the bathwater help heal and tranquilize; a salt rub is cheap and quickly invigorates the skin before any kind of bath.

Apple Cider Vinegar: Combats fatigue and restores the body's natural acid covering.

Sage: Helps stimulate the sweat glands when added to bathwater.

Nutmeg: Can increase perspiration when added to bathwater; also said to be helpful in radiation detoxification.

Rosemary: Stimulates and increases the circulation of the blood.

Pine: Helps to open the pores, soften and stimulate the skin, and cure skin rashes.

Hayflower and Oatstraw: Immediately releases skin impurities.

Bran: Softens the skin.

Fennel and Nettle: Mild detoxifiers.

Epsom Salts: A strong perspiration inducer and muscle relaxer, but it may be too strong for persons in a weakened state.

Ginger Powder Tea and Gingerroot Tea: They relax sore muscles, tone the skin, and greatly improve sluggish circulation. Ginger is so stimulating that it must be used only in small amounts at first, and then gradually increased to your tolerance.

Sulphur: A general healing aid; also helps certain skin problems.

Borax, Starch, and Bicarbonate of Soda: General skin aids.

Dead Sea Salts: Helps restore body functions after injury.

Vitabath and Algemarin: Excellent skin softeners, relaxers, and general body toners.

All of the above are inexpensive and easy to use. The various herbs can be obtained from local health food stores or by mail from botanical suppliers.

Vitabath, Algemarin, pine extract, Dead Sea salts, sulphur, and Aveeno (colloidal oatmeal) are available in drugstores and some department stores.

Never buy too large a quantity of herbs in advance, as they lose their potency in about a year. You can make strong tinctures or extracts of any herb yourself. These will last a very long time, and you can add small amounts of the tincture or extract to the bathwater or compress as needed.

APPLE CIDER VINEGAR BATH

Therapeutic Uses

- Overcome fatigue
- Relieve poison ivy
- Detoxify
- Relieve sunburn
- Relieve itchiness
- Cosmetic for the skin

Apple cider vinegar is a reliable, inexpensive bath aid. I purchase it in quantity so that I never run out and usually transfer the vinegar to decorative flasks and keep one in each bathroom. I add about 1 cup to my bath. But if I am trying to overcome fatigue, I first pour a little of the apple cider vinegar into the cup of my hand and splash it over my shoulders, arms, back, and chest. I then slide into the warm to hot bath and soak with my entire body submerged. Next, I let out the warm water and slowly replace it with cold water, which I splash first over my feet and then sponge over my entire body, allowing it to dribble down my spine. This cold-water splash never fails to invigorate and restore energy.

Add 2 cups of apple cider vinegar to the bathwater to overcome itchiness or relieve poison ivy attacks.

SALT MASSAGE BATH

Therapeutic Uses

- To abort an oncoming cold
- Relieve rheumatism/gout
- Restore circulation

- Add buoyancy
- Overcome sluggishness
- Eliminate dead skin

This is a must when you are feeling low. The salt friction on the body, along with other tonic therapies and relaxing warm baths (filled with herbal substances or coarse salt as described throughout this section), can actually keep you going through stress periods. I always keep a decorative jar of salt on a shelf near my bath so I can make up a quick salt paste for the massage.

Plain coarse salt or sea salt can be used in two different ways or combined into a consecutive treatment. When massaged as a paste over unbroken skin, salt acts as a body stimulant, increases the circulation in anemic conditions, helps to overcome mild depressions, increases the tone of the body before or after an infection, and can help to overcome the body trauma caused by excessive drinking. This massage may be used separately or in combination with an immersion salt bath.

Massage

A vigorous massage with a slushy paste of salt and warm water increases circulation, cleanses the skin and therefore intensifies elimination through the skin, and stimulates both the sebaceous glands and the nervous system. The massage acts as a tonic on the blood vessels and other tissues of the body. The feeling after this rub is one of rejuvenation and renewed vitality.

Sit nude on the edge of a bathtub filled with warm water. Pour a handful of salt into an unbreakable container or the cup of your hand. Add small amounts of water until you have a thick paste. Apply the salt paste in slow, circular motions over the body from the shoulders to the feet. This salt massage may also be applied while you are sitting with both feet in hot water. In this case, also apply a damp cold compress to the forehead.

After the massage, either wash off the salt with a gentle or jet shower, or a cold sponging, or slide into the bath, which you have filled with moderately warm to hot water. Soak the entire body. The massage should only take a few minutes.

Do not use a salt massage if you have skin lesions or inflammation.

SALT BATH

Therapeutic Uses

- To relax
- After too much sitting
- To release tension
- For sluggish skin
- For menopause

Coarse salt can be added to any bath to produce buoyancy, and additional salt may be massaged on the back during the bath. The more salt there is in the water, the greater will be the feeling of relaxation and refreshment.

I find such salt baths, even with only a cup or two of salt, very calming for the body, totally relaxing, and almost hypnotic. The greater the amount of salt, the more you will perspire. Small amounts such as 1 cup do not increase the perspiration. As little as 5 pounds of common coarse salt will approximate natural sea water, which is between 1 percent and 7 percent salt. This acts as a mild tonic on the body in the same way that bathing in the sea creates a feeling of mild euphoria.

I use the combined salt massage and salt bath to overcome sluggishness from sitting at the typewriter most of the day. It is also one of my many weapons to help abort an incipient cold.

Take long salt baths in tepid water whenever possible because the salt holds the heat very well. When a tonic effect is desired, use colder water (75°F to 65°F) and immerse the body for 1 to 2 minutes. End the bath with a cool sponging or a needle shower.

This bath is useful for women in menopause, and for those who need to increase skin activity but whose weakness or cardiac condition do not allow stronger baths.

Algemarin is a sea-algae vitamin foam-bath available in many department stores. It tones, freshens, and revitalizes the body. Dead Sea salts, available in health food stores, also have restorative and softening powers. Both are excellent bath products.

OATMEAL BATH

Therapeutic Uses

- Soothe the skin
- Overcome itchiness
- Overcome hives
- Relieve sunburn, chafing, windburn, dishpan hands

Oatmeal is extraordinary. It is not only useful and dependable in soothing and nourishing the body internally, it also coats, soothes, and restores rough skin. It is a must for baby's bathwater because it overcomes the acidity of urine or diaper rash. It can also be used both as a paste on the body before the bath and in the bathwater to relieve the most stubborn chafing welts between the legs.

Method

To use oatmeal in the bath, either blend raw oatmeal into tiny particles or use a prepared, colloidal, suspended oatmeal. Add up to 1 cup oatmeal to tepid or warm bathwater.

Oatmeal in the bathwater mollifies windburn and sunburn, and relieves itchiness. For treating poison ivy attacks, I alternate between using oatmeal baths with Aveeno (the prepared, colloidal, suspended particles of oatmeal, obtained in the drugstore), and apple cider vinegar baths. Although I prefer using Aveeno, it is quite expensive. You can prepare your own oatmeal body-soother by blending rough cooking oatmeal into a powder. Do this in advance, bottle and label it, and keep in the medicine chest.

HAYFLOWER BATH

Therapeutic Uses

- Detoxify

Hayflower—the very word connotes vast fields of newly grown grass. When I was a child, my family and I collected these flowers, dried them on a huge screen, and stored them in brown paper bags. Sometimes we sewed the hayflowers into minihandkerchief pouches. These we plunged into a quart of boiling water and then poured the extracted "tea" from these pouches into the bathwater whenever we wanted to ease muscular tension, or, especially, to extract toxins before a cold or during an acute bacterial attack. Healthy persons may use this potent extractor as often as they please, but weak or ill persons are advised to use these flowers in moderation. Once a week is often enough for chronic rheumatism or other chronic health problems. See the specific listings in Part 3 for details.

Method

Make a strong tea of the dried hayflowers with about 3 cups of the flowers to 2 quarts of boiling water. Pour the boiling water over the flowers, steep for 15 to 30 minutes, and strain. Add this strained liquid to any partial or full bath. Add tepid, warm, or hot water, depending on the amount of perspiration you wish to induce.

There is an excellent Swiss Alpine Hayflower Bath Extract available from Weleda (see Resources). This is excellent in helping to abort a cold and in overcoming the effects of a poisoned insect bite.

Other Water Therapy Uses for Hayflowers

Hayflowers are frequently yellow, sweet-scented vernal grass; this is the very same grass that gives so much trouble to hay fever victims. You can make a tincture of these hayflowers by soaking them in brandy. A sniff or two in each nostril during a hay fever attack will usually produce instantaneous relief.

Another excellent detoxifying hayflower is the aromatic cleavers, sometimes called goosegrass.

Hayflower compresses or hayflower dipped shirts placed on children will act quickly to bring out the internal eruptions in many children's diseases. See the specific listings in Part 3.

Hayflower arm baths are excellent for any inflammation or wounds on the arms and fingers.

Hayflower footbaths are excellent for any inflammation or wounds on the feet and ankles. They also will help reduce inflammation and pus in the nail bed of the toes, and relieve swelling around open cuts, or tissues filled with blood after an injury. They also help with the problem of sweating feet and they have a remarkable effect on swollen feet.

OATSTRAW BATH

Therapeutic Uses

- Detoxify
- Knots on feet
- Ingrown toenails
- Blisters on the feet
- Sore feet
- Diseases of the bladder
- Sores that turn to pus
- Pain of arthritis, gout, rheumatism

The straw left over when oat is harvested is a very important detoxifying substance. It can be used alone or in combination with hayflowers.

The chemicals in hayflowers can be released by steeping in boiling water, but oatstraw must be simmered for 20 minutes or more. Then steep, strain, and pour into tepid or warm temperature bathwater.

End each bath with a cold sponging and vigorous friction towel rub.

Bladder Problems

For bladder problems take one 10-minute warm oatstraw bath. After a month, plan a series of cold oatstraw baths for several months. Then take the warm baths in the same sequence until the problems are eliminated.

The action of the oatstraw is so strong, it may be debilitating for weak persons.

Foot Problems

Use foot soaks with oatstraw for sore feet, knots on the feet, sores that develop pus, ingrown toenails, and blisters on the feet. Such baths are also useful for the pain of chronic gout, arthritis, and rheumatism.

CHAMOMILE BATH

Therapeutic Uses

- To soothe skin
- To open pores and eliminate blackheads
- As an antiseptic
- For digestive problems
- As a sleeping aid

The mild apple-smelling herb chamomile is one of the most versatile of herbs.

Method

Pour a pint of boiling water over a handful of chamomile flowers in a non-aluminum container, steep for 15 minutes, strain, and pour the strained liquid into a steamy hot bath. Relax in the bath for about 10 minutes. This will open the pores of the body and the face. However, the hot bath will cause lassitude and deplete muscle tone, so end this bath by splashing cold water on your body to restore the tone. Do not use cold water on your face, but as quickly as possible get out of the bath and gently push out facial blackheads with two cotton swabs. (See instructions for chamomile facials on page 142.)

Chamomile helps relieve internal digestive spasms. Add it to the bathwater as above, or pour it on a large, natural sponge and gently massage the abdomen in clockwise, rotating motions. See also the listing of specific problems in Part 3.

PINE BATH

Therapeutic Uses

- Recover after vigorous exercise
- Relax, especially if excessively nervous
- Overcome fatigue
- Relieve breathing problems of asthma, bronchitis
- Increase blood circulation

- Eliminate blackheads
- Increase perspiration

The delightful, heady aroma of pine is available in extract form in several effective products. My favorites are the liquid and/or condensed "tablet" products from the Black Forest of Germany.

Those of you who have had the pleasure of walking through a pine forest will undoubtedly recall the sensation of being able to breathe deeper and lighter. Pine has that kind of effect on the lungs. This in turn gives the kidneys a boost, and they function better.

Method

If the bath is intended to relieve fatigue after exercise or to relax, fill the bathtub with water slightly lower than body temperature, 95°F to 97°F, and pour in one capful of the pine extract. Immerse your entire body. Remain in the bath for 15 to 30 minutes.

If you want to produce sweating, start the bath at the above temperature, add the pine, and increase the hot water to 102°F. Remain in the bath for 10 minutes.

If easing breathing difficulties is the main focus of the bath, take only a partial sit bath. Sit on a rubber pillow placed on the side of the tub. Wear a shirt or wrap a towel over your torso. Use tepid water, and get out of the bath as soon as breathing difficulties are somewhat eased.

In an emergency, if no pine extract is available, you can add 4 ounces of turpentine (a pine product) to the water to aid breathing. However, when using turpentine it is imperative that you keep the genital area out of the bathwater. Do not use turpentine if there are any open sores on the lower part of the body, because the turpentine may irritate the skin.

A small tablet of the concentrated pine extract or a dollop of the green liquified pine added to warm water in the bath reddens the surface of the skin. When blood is drawn to the surface in this type of action, it increases the number of red and white blood cells. Pine also has a special action on the substance cholesterin, which accumulates in the pores of the skin. It is therefore helpful in controlling blackheads.

Pine will increase the tendency of the body to perspire. Run hot water in the bath and add the pine extract according to directions on the bottle or tablet box. The aroma will make the bath feel luxurious, and the pine will relieve muscle fatigue, help in quickly eliminating debris developed during athletic activity, and aid in perspiration (this is especially useful if you are catching a cold).

BRAN BATH

Therapeutic Uses

- Relieve itching
- Invigorate and tone skin and nerves
- Clean surface of skin
- Alleviate nervous conditions

Bran is the outer covering of wheat and is an essential fiber in preventing and overcoming constipation. Bran can be prepared separately and strained before placing in the bathwater, or zipped into close mesh pouches. It makes the water milky white.

Bran has also been used for thousands of years to treat various skin conditions and will help with any generalized itching or dermatitis. It softens the skin and leaves a coating of fine particles on the skin. It can soothe any irritation of the skin. It also subtly eliminates dead skin cells and rough scales.

Bran in the bathwater is useful for nervous conditions, since it helps to invigorate the body and tone up the skin and the nerves at the same time.

Bran can be added to several alkaline substances, such as sodium bicarbonate and borax for antiseptic purposes, and starch for cooling the skin and allaying itching, chafing, poison ivy, and eczema.

Method

Sew several handfuls of bran into a cheesecloth pouch. Soak in very hot water for several minutes. Fill the bathtub with neutral water—slightly under body temperature (96°F). Place the pouch in the water and squeeze it until the water turns milky white.

Another method is slightly messier, but has a wonderful effect on certain dermatological problems. Cover the faucet with the bran cheesecloth pouch and fill the bathtub with warm water. Get in. While the bath is filling, sponge your body with hot water. Remove the cheesecloth. The bran friction rub invigorates and soothes.

Always finish a bran bath with vigorous towel rub of the body. If you can, allow the fine particles of bran to stay on the body. If you prefer, you may sponge them off with tepid or cool water.

Water Temperature: 95°F to 98°F.

Duration: Bran baths can last from a half-hour up to several hours, if desired.

CORNSTARCH, BORAX, SODIUM BICARBONATE BATHS

Therapeutic Uses

- To soothe skin
- As an antiseptic

Several household products can be added to the bath. Cornstarch is an excellent dusting powder that absorbs excess perspiration. When added to the bath, it is also an effective cooling agent. Used alone or with bran or oatmeal, it moderates the itchiness of poison ivy, poison oak, eczema, and prickly heat. Add between 1 cup and 1 pound of cornstarch to a warm bath.

Borax is an antiseptic that makes the bathwater soft and slippery and the body feel very pleasant. It tends to be slightly drying, however. For the full effect, add between ½ to 1 cup to warm bathwater.

The 1887 *United States Dispensatory* notes that some physicians were successful in treating ringworm of the scalp with a borax-vinegar wash. This consisted of a large pinch of borax plus 2 ounces of distilled vinegar. Combine the items in larger proportions for a bath for ringworm patients.

Sodium bicarbonate in the bathwater opens the pores, cleanses the body, acts as a mild antiseptic, and relieves itching and skin irritation. Use from half a pound to a pound in neutral-temperature water.

EPSOM SALT BATH

Therapeutic Uses

- Increase perspiration

- Relieve neuritis, lumbago, arthritis, sciatica, rheumatism
- Abort an illness
- Eliminate toxic debris
- Relieve muscular fatigue
- Help control catarrh

Epsom salts added to hot bathwater will induce profuse perspiration. This bath should be used particularly before the onset of a cold, flu, or other infection. Such baths are also helpful in relaxing the body after strenuous exercise, and for pain relief in chronic arthritis, sciatica, and rheumatism. However, these baths tend also to deplete the body, so do not take them if you are weak or have heart trouble, arteriosclerosis, diabetes, or are postoperative. Also, Epsom salts are very potent and may bother some people.

Method

Put protective material such as a rubber sheet or an old wool blanket on the bed.

Fill the tub with hot water to your utmost temperature tolerance. Dissolve from 1 cup to 1 pound of the Epsom salts. The more salts, the more perspiration. Before entering the tub, apply the first of several consecutive large cold compresses to the forehead and head, and then sit submerged in the hot water for 10 to 20 minutes. While in the tub, drink a hot herbal tea—peppermint, thyme, sage, etc.—or some other fluid to further increase perspiration and replace lost fluids.

The length of time you stay in the bath depends on your age and health, but since the heat and the perspiration tend to be weakening, no matter what age you are, get out of the bath slowly.

Do not dry yourself, but cover your body with large towels and go to bed immediately. Lie under a coverlet and allow body perspiration to continue. If you fall asleep, wait until morning to sponge off with tepid water. Conclude the wash with a cool-water sponging and a vigorous rub to dry the body. If you do not fall asleep after half an hour or so, sponge off as above and dry vigorously. Then change the bedclothes, go back to bed, and enjoy a long, restful sleep.

SULPHUR BATH

Therapeutic Uses

- Relieve skin ailments
- Relieve pain of arthritis, chronic gout, neuritis
- Heal the body
- Overcome acne
- Mild antiseptic
- Mild antiparasite

Natural sulphur waters have helped patients to overcome a wide variety of skin ailments and to heal the body internally as well as externally.

Method

Fill the bathtub with tepid water and add from $\frac{1}{2}$ to $1\frac{1}{2}$ cups of colloidal (fine suspended particles) sulphur or a sulphur-bath preparation. Sit submerged in the bath for 10 to 20 minutes. The sulphur is reduced chemically to sulphurated hydrogen, which when absorbed by the skin has a great healing, cleansing, and antiseptic effect.

Sulphur baths are also helpful for treating acne.

Water Temperature: 95°F to 102°F.

ASCORBIC ACID BATH

Therapeutic Uses

- Allergy attack
- Hemorrhoids
- Infection

I would never have thought of using ascorbic acid powder (vitamin C) in the bath, except that on a hunch I poured 3 tablespoons in a warm bath during a sudden allergy attack. Shortly after this, to my amazement, the sneezing stopped altogether!

Dr. John Hanks, athletic consultant for the Denver Broncos and Denver Nuggets, who is also a proponent of water therapy, recommends using ascorbic acid sit baths (shallow baths) to treat hemorrhoids. Hemorrhoids are a problem that afflict many athletes and dancers, and Dr. Hanks feels that the addition of ascorbic acid to the bath greatly speeds up the healing process. Add 1 cup of the powder to 5 quarts of cool water (the water should be as cool as you can tolerate). Sit in the bath for 3 to 15 minutes, depending on your tolerance.

SHAMPOO

Therapeutic Uses

- Clean hair
- Clean body
- Clean scalp
- Increase skin action
- Overcome energy blocks
- Stimulate acupuncture pressure points
- Detoxify

Did you ever stop to think why you feel so good after you take a cleansing bath and shampoo your hair? Shampooing with water, a good emollient, nondetergent soap, and hand pressure or friction materials not only cleanses and refreshes the body, but eliminates dead skin cells and opens the pores of the skin. This helps to pass unneeded material out of the system. A shampoo also stimulates the internal organs—acting like an electric light switch in "turning on" crucial hand, foot, face, and scalp pressure points. This is why a strong hair wash and scalp rub (with careful drying) can sometimes turn the tide in eliminating a head cold.

When you shampoo, the protective acid mantle of the skin is gradually washed away. It is necessary to restore this acid barrier. I do this by using diluted apple cider vinegar as one of my restorative hair rinses.

There are many fine herbal shampoos and soaps on the market. Many are made from pure products that will heal the body, tone up the skin, soften the skin, and also restore the pH balance. In addition to the excellent products found in most health food stores today, the following are some of my favorite mail-order firms: Caswell-Massey has a truly international selection of interesting shampoos and soaps. The Weleda Company manufactures and imports Swiss and German bath products, including a great chestnut shampoo, which is useful if you have hard water. Culpeper The Herbalist is a chain of stores in Great Britain, started by the Society of Herbalists, that sell very high-quality shampoos and soaps (I like the cucumber and almond oil products). Another unusual mail-order source is D. Napier's and Sons of Edinburgh. This organization of family herbalists opened its doors in 1860 and manufactures a very healing, emollient slippery elm soap. (See Resources.)

SHAMPOO FOR HAIR

You should choose a shampoo and rinse that suit your hair texture and will restore its pH balance. Dry, normal, and oily hair all need a different shampoo and rinse. It therefore pays to experiment with the different natural-based shampoos on the market. Do not use a regular cake soap as a shampoo—it will dull the hair. And be wary of the highly promoted anti-dandruff shampoos. They contain chemicals that can sometimes irritate. In general, proper scalp stimulation, frequent brushing, cleansing with a mild shampoo, and taking appropriate amounts of vitamins, exercise, rest, and sunshine will make the skin and hair lustrous and healthy.

If you have a chronic disease condition, you should wash your hair and scalp frequently in order to stimulate circulation and eliminate toxins from the body.

SHAMPOO FOR BODY

If you go to a spa or an old-fashioned Turkish bath you will be lathered from head to toe with soap, and a skilled practitioner will scrub your body with a large scrubbing brush. The scrubbing stimulates your body so that you will feel tingly and wide awake. After the scrub you will shower—always ending with cold water. Then you will be encouraged to take a short nap. Because of the exhilarating scrub, you will fall asleep instantly and awaken totally refreshed.

This body shampoo can be somewhat duplicated at home. Begin by soaking the body in a vegetable oil (olive oil is preferred). Soak in a bathtub full of warm to hot water. Soap the body completely with a natural, non-detergent, hard-milled soap, and scrub with a loofah, an aloe brush, a natural bristle brush, or a hand-crocheted Israeli or Mexican hemp washcloth. Scrub gently at first, then work up to a vigorous scrubbing. If the skin is very delicate or sensitive, use a large natural sponge for the first few weeks and then graduate to the friction mitt or brush.

Other shampoos may be preceded with a salt massage to increase circulation.

End each bath with cool to cold water, especially on the feet. Splash apple cider vinegar or diluted apple cider vinegar and rose water over the body. For a truly exhilarating feeling, use the Scots shower—alternate long hot and short cold streams. Vigorously rub the body dry.

PACKS

*P*acks are an ancient concept. Water and cloths have long been used to create and to develop specific states in the body. Each step of these procedures should be done cautiously. Test and check each step to ensure safety.

DAMP COLD SHEET PACK (COLD DOUBLE BODY COMPRESS)

Therapeutic Uses

- Fever
- Muscular problems
- Children's diseases
- Menopause heat
- Nervousness
- Oncoming cold or flu
- As a tonic
- As a sedative
- As an eliminative

- Skin diseases
- Joint problems

This pack is the most effective and powerful of all the water therapies.

Although the directions for this pack may seem complicated at first, it is actually only a long, double body compress that separates the legs by a layer of cloth. This pack is exceptional in helping to overcome fevers. A three-quarter or half pack may be used several times a day. It is also very helpful for most chronic diseases, in detoxifying the body and for aborting an oncoming flu or cold attack.

The action of this compress or body pack is like that of a giant detoxifying magnet. For this reason, except in the case of fever, do not use it too often. Do not use this technique after meals. (See "Cold Double Compress" section for three-quarter and half trunk or smaller packs.)

Method

1. Prepare a hot water bottle. Protect the bed by covering it with two large blankets, their ends lower than the sides of the bed. Then place a large, dry white sheet on top of the blankets. You will later lay a cold wet sheet on top of the dry sheet. The hot water bottle will warm the feet.
2. Have a perspiration-inducing drink, such as peppermint, hayflower, or oatstraw tea, ready at the bedside and by the bath.
3. Have containers of cold water for the cold compress at bath and bedside.
4. Prepare the damp wet sheet by plunging a large white cotton cloth or sheet into cold water. Wring it out so that it is damp, but not too wet. Keep it in the sink to apply directly after the bath while you are standing, or place it on the bed on the dry sheet for when you emerge from the bath.
5. Prepare a full hot bath or a hot footbath. A full hot bath is preferred for total relaxation, sedation, and perspiration induction. You can increase the detoxification effect by adding up to 5 cups of Epsom salts, 1 cup of pine extract, 1 cup of hayflower tea, or 1 tablespoon of hayflower extract to the bathwater.
6. Void the bladder.

7. If you are trying to abort a cold or the flu, consider also taking a cold water enema before the bath.

8. Apply a cold compress to the forehead. Enter the hot bath or take a hot footbath (see pages 85–93). Drink herbal drinks. The bath may last from 15 to 30 minutes depending on your comfort and vitality. (Hot baths tend to sap the energy from the body.) Perspiration starts.

9. Get out of the bath.

10. There are two methods of wrapping. The shortcut is to lift your hands and wrap the cold damp sheet around your body. Wrap some towels around your body, go to the bed, discard the towels, and lie down. Separate your limbs. Then wrap the dry sheet and blankets around your body.

11. The "authentic" method is to first place the wet sheet from the sink on the bed before going into the bath. Then wrap your body in large towels, put on slippers, discard the towels, and quickly lie down on the bed on the cold damp sheet with your arms upraised. As rapidly as possible, bring the right half of the wet sheet over the trunk and right leg. Tuck it in, and lay the loose folds between the legs. Lower the arms. Bring the left half of the sheet over the front of your body. Cover your shoulders, trunk, arms, and left leg. Turn on your left side, and the sheet goes under the right side. Turn up any excess.

Pin the cotton sheet so that no air can emerge. It should be snug, but not tight. Do not let two skin surfaces touch. The sheet is between the skin and the blanket. Next, fold the blankets snugly over your body in envelope fashion.

If you feel feeble, place a hot water bottle on your feet to speed the reaction. Additional light covers may also be added to speed the reaction. They can be applied from chin to ankles, but do not cover the feet. Tuck them in around the shoulders, and remove extra blankets as soon as the heat reaction occurs.

For very nervous persons who cannot bear the thought of being wrapped up, use a less extensive pack up to the armpits. The arms are left free. This three-quarter or half pack will have many of the same results as the full pack. If you have no heat reaction or get cold, take the pack off, cover yourself, and place hot water bottles at your feet.

During a high fever, leave the pack on for 10 to 30 minutes and reapply it later. If you are using the pack to relieve excessive menopausal heat, leave it on for 20 minutes to several hours. The pack may be left on overnight, particularly when you are attempting to avert a potential illness.

If you are using this pack to overcome the flu, an optional step is to "paint" the soles of the feet with liquified garlic tea that has been added to some heavy cold cream or Vaseline. Then put white cotton socks on your feet and put your feet under the wet sheet, covered by the dry sheet and the blankets.

End the application by sponging your body with diluted apple cider vinegar. Do this in sections so that you do not become chilled. Dry, using a coarse towel. Change the bed linens.

Since this is a perspiration-inducing technique and is not energizing, you should then go back to bed. Sip diluted apple cider vinegar and water; apple juice; equal amounts of apple cider vinegar and honey (1 to 3 tablespoons) and a cup of water; or, if desired, any vegetable juice obtained by extraction. If you are very sick, stick to only one type of juice during the day, as a mono diet will speed the healing.

HOT MOIST PACK OR HOT BLANKET PACK

Therapeutic Uses

- Chronic joint and muscular rheumatism
- Sciatica
- Kidney stones
- Nephritis (not as good as hot half baths)
- Blood poisoning
- Children's diseases
- Children's convulsions
- To create profuse perspiration
- To elevate body temperature
- Gout
- Chronic neuralgia
- Mental disturbances

This pack is applied in the same way as the damp sheet pack except that the cotton or linen sheet or preferably blanket is plunged into 110°F hot water. Wring dry, because a very wet blanket loses heat too quickly.

Similar hot packs can be devised for any area of the body. These partial packs help to shunt blood into other areas to break up congestion.

The value of the hot moist pack is that it induces perspiration very quickly, and thus helps eliminate toxic material through the skin. It also decreases internal congestion. Cotton and linen packs are used for children and feeble persons, but blankets retain the heat longer than a cotton sheet and can be used whenever sustained heat action is needed.

The warm moist pack was used by Dr. J. H. Kellogg to hasten the release of toxins in sick children. He considered it more valuable than any drug.

Method

1. Prepare an ice bag, several hot water bottles, and a blanket or sheet to steep in the hot water.
2. Prepare the bed with protective material. It is useful, but not entirely necessary, to first use a rubber or plastic sheet. Over this, place two small blankets or one very large blanket. The blanket should be large enough to overlap the edge of the bed, reach to your neck, and still have room at the bottom to turn up like an envelope.
3. Use either a large cotton or linen sheet, or an old soft wool blanket. Fold the blanket or sheet in thirds, then lengthwise. Holding the ends, immerse it into an extremely hot water bath. Use rubber gloves to wring or squeeze out all of the water.
4. Place the wrung-out blanket or sheet over the dry blankets on the bed, and lie on the bed on your back with arms upraised.
5. Apply a cold compress to the forehead and place an ice bag wrapped in a dish towel on your heart.
6. Wrap the wet blanket over the right side of your body. Bring your arms down and quickly drape the left side of the wet blanket over the front of the body.
7. Wrap the dry blanket(s) over the wet one, tucking it in at the shoulders and the feet. If there is a large rubber or plastic sheet underneath the dry blankets, bring it up and tuck it in at this time (it will help retain the heat longer and cause additional perspiration).
8. Place a series of hot water bottles at the feet and along the sides of the body.

9. Drink copious amounts of water or herb drinks.
10. Continuously replace the forehead compress so that it is always cold.

This pack can be applied for 5 to 20 minutes, depending on your health. The results are so pleasant that you will want to repeat it often, but too many treatments will make you feel exhausted.

There is a danger of becoming chilled when the covers are removed, so remove them in the following manner. Slide out the hot water bottles, the ice bag, the wet blankets and rubber sheet, and have a helper slide in a large dry, warm sheet. Make sure you are continuously covered with the dry blanket. Rub the warm sheet gently over your entire body to get dry. Replace this sheet (it will be damp) with a dry one. Apply another hot water bottle to the feet. Rest or sleep for several hours.

This pack relaxes and soothes the muscles and helps to eliminate toxins and eruptions. It does, however, increase the body temperature and the pulse rate. The pulse rate must be watched—especially with children and feeble persons. If it increases too rapidly, end the procedure. Heart patients, diabetics, persons with arteriosclerosis or TB, or excessively feeble or aged persons should not use this pack.

DRY BLANKET PACK

Therapeutic Uses

- To induce perspiration
- For chronic rheumatism
- In coma
- In shock
- In collapse after hemorrhage

The dry blanket pack is Preissnitz's original preparation for creating perspiration and inducing the elimination of liquids. It is an indispensable aid in reviving someone from a coma, and a valuable therapy for chronic rheumatism (the dry pack, unlike the hot moist pack, does not make you feel weak). This very simple wrapping produces a powerful reaction.

Method

Prepare the bed with two blankets, one on top of the other. If desired, a dry sheet can be placed on top.

Prepare a hot water bottle. This is especially useful for feeble patients or those who will need a boost in heating the body.

Prepare hot lemonade or any of these hot herbal teas: peppermint, thyme, sage, red raspberry. Small amounts of yarrow may be added. Use $1/8$ to $1/4$ teaspoon of cayenne pepper tea added to 1 cup of boiling water to help control internal hemorrhaging.

Void the bladder.

Take a 15- to 30-minute hot bath or hot footbath. Apply a cold compress to the forehead.

Tuck the blanket (or if a sheet is also used, tuck the sheet and then the blanket) around the body. To increase perspiration, apply hot water bottles to the soles of the feet and the sides of the body.

Rest in a warm, well-ventilated room for a half-hour. If there is a free flow of perspiration, apply a cold compress to the head.

Sponge the body with cold water, or immerse the entire body in a full cold bath for 30 seconds to 1 minute. Vigorously dry the body with a large coarse towel and go back to bed. A refreshing sleep follows quickly, symptoms lessen, and you will generally show a marked improvement.

Do not use the pack if eruptive diseases (measles, scarlet fever, chicken pox, and the like), diabetes, arteriosclerosis, or cardiac weakness are present, or if you are excessively nervous.

MUSTARD PACK OR PLASTER

Therapeutic Uses

- Break up internal congestion
- Relieve pain
- Lumbago
- Neuritis
- Improve local circulation
- Bronchitis
- Sciatica

- Act as counterirritant
- Alleviate gout

This is one of my favorite plant packs. Mustard powder (plus a touch of water and flour), when made into a paste and applied in a cloth on a lightly oiled skin, has the power to bring blood to the surface of the skin. It quickly heats up the area, and as the blood rushes to the skin surface, even the worst congestion diminishes.

Method

Prepare some paper toweling and a large linen or cotton dish towel. Fold the cloth in thirds. In a bowl, mix 1 tablespoon of dry, powdered (not hot) mustard with 4 to 8 tablespoons of flour. The less flour, the stronger the effect. To make the pack stronger, use equal amounts of mustard and flour. Double and triple the amounts according to the size of poultice needed. Moisten the mixture with tepid water (hot water prevents the release of the needed oils) until it has the consistency of cream cheese.

Place the mustard paste on the paper toweling. Fold the toweling to make a packet, and place it in the folded dish cloth or clean folded cotton cloth. Heat the pack by placing it on a hot water bottle.

If you have sensitive skin, oil the skin lightly with olive or vegetable oil. Place a thin cloth such as a large man's handkerchief on the area. Apply the mustard pack (or plaster). Cover the area with a blanket.

At first the heat may seem intense, but then it lessens, and in my experience, always seems merely hot. As the skin becomes very red, the pack can be transferred from area to area, from the front of the chest to the upper back (for bronchitis) or on areas of intense pain.

Apply the pack to each area for 2 to 10 minutes. The entire treatment should last a half-hour. After this, the pack loses its potency.

EARTH PACKS

Therapeutic Uses

- Rheumatic problems
- Neuralgia
- Pain

- Arthritis
- Muscle spasms
- Chronic joint inflammation
- Chronic sciatica
- Burns
- Stings
- To neutralize toxins
- Gout

Hot sand, hot mud packs, and clay packs have been used for centuries by different cultures to relieve joint pain. The material used is either organic volcanic ash, peat from bogs, mineral sea mud, or clay from high mineral areas. All of these substances are available in powder form. For ordinary household first aid, I keep an inexpensive 5-pound ball of neutral Jordan clay ready in a closed container.

Clay packs have extracting ability because the mineral content increases the heat and chemical action on the skin. Because clay and/or earth draw out poisons, such packs not only soften the skin and release tension around joints, but also absorb internal toxic or pathogenic material.

The Cattier Company of France makes several excellent, neutral green-clay products including powdered green clay, clay toothpaste, clay soap, and clay masks. Weleda sells an excellent internal and external clay (Luvos #1, #2). Pottery firms, or firms that service rehabilitation departments of hospitals or spas, may be a source of other therapeutic earth substances.

Method

Heat up the clay or mud in a large double boiler. Add pure mineral or spring water to soften it. Spread it in 1- or 2-inch thicknesses on a soft cotton cloth, slightly larger than the area you wish to cover. Place the hot clay or mud directly on the hurt area. Cover the area with a dry lightweight cloth. Leave on until it dries (15 to 30 minutes). Rinse off with warm water, then splash with a little cool water.

When an area is inflamed or hot, as in a burn, use cold "chunks" of moistened clay to extract the heat. Envelop the area in a thick layer of wet clay, and the pain will seem to disappear. Next, cover the area with plastic or oilskin to keep it moist.

In the case of a severe burn, however, it is imperative to see a physician.

Earth packs can also be made by adding layer upon layer of the hot (or cold) clay directly on the skin. Or the hot "mud" can be placed in a small cotton pillowcase with an "open window" and applied directly to the area. I used just such an application of cold mud to neutralize and detoxify my body during a case of food poisoning.

Small applications of clay or mud will revitalize almost any area, but do not take large baths in mud if you have heart disease, diabetes, high blood pressure, or arteriosclerosis.

SHOWERS

A shower is a directed stream of water used on one area or the whole body. The temperature, shape, and force of each shower determines its healing and physiological effects.

Showers can be rain or fan (gentle, dispersed stream with low pressure), or jet or percussion (powerful, direct stream with great pressure). They are used at cold, hot, neutral, or alternating temperatures. A dousing shower is one poured from a pail or a great height.

COLD SHOWER

Therapeutic Uses

- As a tonic
- To overcome fatigue
- To reduce high temperatures
- To overcome collapse

Use water that is as cold as you can tolerate. Remain in the shower for at least several seconds. Your endurance to the cold will increase as you do this regularly.

HOT SHOWER

Therapeutic Uses

- Prepare a patient for a cold treatment
- Sedate central nervous system
- Soothe irritated skin
- Alleviate pain

A light rain shower eases neuralgic pains and alleviates the discomfort of hives and itching. During a very hot shower, prevent headache or dizziness by applying a cold compress on the forehead and neck.

Water Temperature: 100°F to 104°F.
Duration: 30 seconds to 2 minutes.

NEUTRAL SHOWER

Therapeutic Uses

- Pelvic problems
- Nervousness
- Bedwetting

A light, gentle fan or spray shower in lukewarm, body-temperature water will relax and calm the body by contracting the brain's blood vessels. It acts in the same way as a long neutral bath. Neutral showers are useful for seminal weakness, bedwetting, and some cases of painful vaginal spasm.

Water Temperature: 92°F to 97°F.
Duration: 4 to 6 minutes.

ALTERNATE HOT AND COLD SHOWER

Because of their varied uses, alternate hot and cold applications may be the most important of the healing showers. There are two types of alternate hot and cold showers: equal amounts of hot and cold water and unequal amounts, with emphasis on the hot stream.

EQUAL: ALTERNATE HOT AND COLD

Therapeutic Uses

- Muscular rheumatism
- Stiff joints (if no inflammation of nerves)
- Enlargement of liver

Direct water on body or local area.

Duration: 15 seconds hot, then 15 seconds cold.

UNEQUAL: LONGER HOT, SHORTER COLD (SCOTS SHOWER)

Therapeutic Uses for the Whole Body

- Muscle fatigue
- Lack of energy
- Profuse or frequent sweating

Therapeutic Uses for Localized Areas of the Body

- Poor circulation
- Chronic backache
- Spinal irritations
- Uterine and ovarian neuralgia
- Gastric ulcer
- Congestion of the brain (when used on feet alone)

This is my favorite of all showers, for it has a remarkable and tonic effect on the body. This Scots shower is excellent for the circulation, and when used over a long period of time tends to affirm circulatory changes. It achieves the circulatory effect of an extreme, short cold-water treatment without producing any internal heat reaction within the body.

Use the hot jet spray for 1 to 4 minutes. Follow immediately with a cold jet spray for 5 to 30 seconds.

If the cold spray is used for less than 10 seconds (but no less than 5 seconds), the general effect is one of increased circulation and sedation.

If the cold spray is used for more than 10 seconds (but no longer than 30 seconds), the body feels tonified and stimulated.

SPECIAL USES OF UNEQUAL ALTERNATE HOT AND COLD SHOWERS

Therapeutic Uses

- Dry skin
- Profuse sweating
- Gastrointestinal catarrh
- Congestion of liver and spleen
- Chronic gastritis
- Cardiac inefficiency
- Inflammation of uterus

Use streams of warm to hot water on areas that need stimulation. Gradually increase the heat, depending on your tolerance.

Use heat for 1 to 2 minutes or until the skin is cherry colored. Follow with the cold spray for 2 to 3 seconds.

LOCAL SHOWERS

Local showers directed to only one part of the body can affect other parts of the body by reflex, or by diverting blood from that area.

SOLES OF FEET

Therapeutic Uses

- Cold feet

- Ejaculation of sperm because of relaxed condition
- Weakness of bladder
- Incontinence in the elderly

Use the strong cold jet stream for $\frac{1}{2}$ minute to 2 minutes.

ENTIRE FOOT

Therapeutic Uses

- Prevents headaches

A cold broken jet or spray shower on the feet at the end of any shower contracts the blood vessels of the brain and relieves any congestion in the head.

ABDOMEN

COLD

Therapeutic Uses

- Constipation
- Dilation of the colon
- Pelvic displacement caused by weakness

Duration: A few seconds.

HOT

Therapeutic Uses

- Pain and irritability in the bladder, uterus, ovaries, and pelvic area

Duration: 3 to 5 minutes.

ALTERNATE HOT AND COLD

Therapeutic Uses

- Relieve irritation in lower back

- Tone abdominal organs
- Help overcome chronic diarrhea

Duration: 3 minutes hot; 30 seconds cold. Repeat several times.

FAN SPRAY SHOWER TO CHEST

COLD

Therapeutic Uses

- To top, side, or back of chest: Increase flow of blood to skin, muscles, and lungs
- To breast: Stimulate blood to pelvis, contract muscles of uterus

Duration: A few seconds.

PROLONGED COLD

Therapeutic Uses

- To chest: Contract blood vessels of lungs, lessen blood to lungs
- To breast: Contract blood vessels of uterus and relieve uterine congestion
- To breastbone (lower sternum): Contract kidney blood vessels, increase flow of urine

Duration: 2 minutes.

JET SHOWER TO SHOULDER

Therapeutic Uses

- Delay in development of young women
- Absence or abnormal stopping of menstrual period
- Constipation
- Bladder troubles
- Incontinence

A short cold shoulder shower (1 minute) followed by a 3-minute very hot shower (113°F and up) acts on the pelvic area and all other lower extremities through reflex action.

FACE AND SCALP

An application of very cold water on any part of the skin produces an excitant effect on the brain. A prolonged cold shower relieves congestion; a short cold shower increases activity in the area. A neutral face and scalp shower relieves tension and excitement.

UPWARD PELVIC FLOOR AND ANUS

To obtain bidet attachments for upward showers, do a search on the Internet to find a supplier.

COLD

Therapeutic Uses

- To anus only: Useful for hemorrhoids and constipation
- For women: Upward shower acts on bladder, fallopian tubes
- For men: Upward shower acts on prostate, ejaculatory ducts, testicles, bladder, pelvis, deep urethra

HOT

Therapeutic Uses

- Rectal ulcers, fissures

End a hot upward shower with several seconds of cold spray.

DOUSING SHOWER

Therapeutic Uses

- High fevers
- Sunstroke

- Hysteria
- Agitation of mentally disturbed
- Children's diseases (when air passages are clogged)
- Scarlatina (scarlet fever)
- Asphyxiation

Pouring cold water over the body sharply awakens the vital forces. Such a shower is excellent for eliminating unnatural body heat (from fever and sunstroke) and for stimulating breathing. If you are treating someone who is in an alcoholic stupor, make sure to rub the body afterward with a towel to avoid secondary complications. If the skin of the person you are treating is exceptionally cold (as with nearly drowned persons), apply a hot water bottle or hot water to get the body more active.

A neutral temperature dousing that is directed to the spine, arm, foot, or feet has a sedative effect.

Do not use dousing if there are heart or kidney problems, or if there is any internal bleeding.

Method

Have a large sheet ready for rubbing the body. This is very important, both to sharpen the effect of the application and to avoid secondary complications.

Wrap a cold towel around the patient's head. Pour water from as great a height as possible. The patient can stand or sit in the tub with hands crossed over the chest. The treatment can also be combined with the patient sitting in a hot water bath. Direct the first pailful of water to the chest, the second to the back. Rub trunk and limbs with a large dry sheet for 20 seconds. Wrap the patient in the sheet and rub until the entire body is dry.

ENEMA

An enema is an injection of water into the rectum.

Therapeutic Uses

- Eject waste materials from the lower bowel
- Evacuate fecal material from the lower colon

- Create kidney activity in disease states
- Lower the temperature in fever
- Stimulate the liver
- Relieve irritation or pain in rectum
- Relieve inflammation in rectum
- Control diarrhea
- Help with painful menstrual periods
- Reduce pain in acute pelvic conditions
- Reduce abdominal inflammation
- Relieve cystitis

Method

To use such an irrigation, obtain a rubber gravity (fountain) syringe from a drugstore. Close the valve controlling the tube and fill with several cups of water. Warm water is used in most evacuations, cold water is used in fever, and hot water is used to stimulate the body during certain health problems or diseases. Use 2 pints of water for adults; $\frac{1}{2}$ to 1 pint for children, according to age. Five tablespoons of pure, undiluted coffee added to 1 quart of water is detoxifying and may be used when necessary. Chamomile tea will help reduce internal spasms. Catnip tea will relieve spasms and constipation.

Attach the rubber bottle to a hook about $4\frac{1}{2}$ to 5 feet high on the wall or on the bathroom door. Lubricate the nozzle with cream, but make sure to keep the nozzle holes open. Although an enema may be taken while sitting upright on the toilet, the best position is the knee-to-chest position on the floor. This changes the entire position of the bowel and colon, and water can penetrate into the body for quite a distance. If it is more convenient, take the enema while lying on the floor on your left side.

Insert the nozzle into the rectum, open the pressure clip, eliminate the air, and allow the water to flow into the body. Try not to let in air, as this can be uncomfortable. Stop the water flow by pinching the rubber tube. Rub your abdomen in a clockwise fashion. This allows you to retain the water comfortably for a longer period of time.

Hot rectal irrigation is useful for painful cystitis, rectal spasm, rectal pain, hemorrhoidal pain, for expelling gas or controlling gas, and for relieving pelvic pain. It will stimulate kidney function even when all drugs fail. Cold enemas stimulate the bowel profoundly and can be used to shrink hemorrhoids, help reduce fever, and help the body throw off a cold.

In treating chronic colitis, use a honey or molasses enema for its purging effect in reducing mucus and loosening hardened accumulations of mucus.

Enemas must not be used too often, or the body will lose its tone and ability to evacuate normally. When traveling or for postoperative constipation, Fleet enemas can be used. They are available in sizes for adults and children and can be purchased at drugstores.

VAGINAL DOUCHE

A vaginal douche is an irrigation of the vaginal area with water or a medicated remedy, such as rosemary tea.

Therapeutic Uses

- Relieve itching
- Relieve spasm
- Relieve pain
- Overcome yeast infection
- Help control pain or flow before period
- Overcome white discharge

Purchase a special hand vaginal spray or use the long spray nozzle available with all fountain syringes. This can be attached to a wall. The water flows in by gravity.

Method

Fill the bag with plain water or medicated water as described under "Vaginal Problems," pages 279–281. Sit on the toilet or in the bathtub and let the water flow in and out of the bulb syringe or nozzle.

Weak rosemary tea douches can be used for a week or so to overcome many vaginal and ovarian problems. Use 1 tablespoon to 1 cup of boiling water. Steep the rosemary for 20 minutes, strain, and add to a quart-sized douche bag.

Normally, the vaginal cavity should not be douched too often, because irrigation eliminates normal body acidity.

How to Classify Water Temperature

	Fahrenheit	Centigrade
Very cold	32°–56°	0°–13.3°
Cold	56°–65°	13.3°–18.3°
Cool	65°–75°	18.3°–23.9°
Tepid	75°–92°	23.9°–33.3°
Neutral	92°–98°	33.3°–36.1°
Warm to hot	98°–104°	36.1°–40°
Very hot	104° and above	40° and above

When You Don't Have a Thermometer

For a hot bath you will need 1 quart of very hot or boiling water for every 2 quarts of cold water. Place the cold water in the bath first and add the hot water in order not to lose the heat. Use the same proportion for gallons of water.

Cold Water (53°F)	Boiling Water (212°F)	Bathwater
2 quarts	1 quart	3 quarts 106°F
2½ quarts	1 quart	3½ quarts 98°F
3 quarts	1 quart	4 quarts 93°F
4 quarts	1 quart	5 quarts 85°F
5 quarts	1 quart	6 quarts 80°F

continued on next page

WHEN YOU DON'T HAVE A THERMOMETER *continued*

| 6 quarts | 1 quart | 7 quarts 76°F |
| 8 quarts | 1 quart | 9 quarts 71°F |

To gradually increase the water temperature of a bath, remove 1 cup of the bathwater and add 2 cups of very hot or boiling water. Each replacement increases the bath temperature by 1°F.

STEAM

*T*he gaseous state of water is produced by heating water to a high temperature. The wet or dry (sauna) steam is invaluable in stimulating the skin, and the resultant perspiration helps to evacuate stored toxins. However, since the water must be hot before it turns to steam, it must be handled very cautiously. Test and check each step of these suggested procedures to ensure personal safety.

VAPORIZER BATH

Therapeutic Uses

- Open pores
- Open clogged nostrils
- Relieve head cold
- Relieve sinus attack
- Help breathing problems
- Relieve bronchitis
- Restore voice, overcome hoarseness and laryngitis

Use the steam from a boiling kettle, an electric home vaporizer, or a cold steam humidifier. An 8-hour electric steam vaporizer is a useful home item because it brings moist air into dry, overheated, winterized rooms and facilitates breathing for all chest and sinus conditions, as well as for those with colds whose nostrils are clogged. It is a big help in a house with children.

Method

Add a few drops of compound or simple tincture of benzoin to the vaporizer lid. The tincture is made from a resin, so it will leave a gummy film, but it is very helpful for chest complaints and has the added advantage of being a cosmetic aid. It is also a remarkable aid in restoring the voice.

If no electric vaporizer is available, boil water in a kettle and keep it going by means of an electric tray, or some other safe arrangement. Create an improvised tent over your body and direct the steam so that you don't get too wet or perspired. A large umbrella can be used. Occasionally sponge yourself or use a cold mitten massage on your body. This will aid circulation and give a feeling of well-being.

FACIALS

To duplicate a professional facial, bring to a vigorous boil in a Pyrex pot 2 quarts of water to which 2 tablespoons of chamomile tea have been added. Remove the pot from the heat, place a newspaper on a table, and place the hot pot on the paper. Sit with your face above the pot (but not close enough to get burned). Improvise a tent by covering your head and the pot with a towel so that no steam escapes. Sit under the "tent" with eyes closed for 5 to 10 minutes, breathing with your mouth open. The pores of the face will open, and perspiration will pour out. Afterward, gently push out the blackheads with a cotton swab. This procedure is most useful for those with excessively oily skin. Do this in a nondrafty area to avoid being chilled. Close the pores with a splash of cool water and sweep the face with a cotton pad moistened with an herbal astringent, such as witch hazel.

HOME STEAM BATH

Therapeutic Uses

- Arthritis
- Fractures
- Gout
- Sprains
- Sciatica
- Chronic low back pain
- Before tonic cold therapy to eliminate stored toxins
- To create perspiration

A free flow of perspiration will often relieve the extreme pain of arthritis, gout, or sciatica, and ease other pain. Steam baths are often available in local gyms, and are now available in steamroom or prebuilt sauna units for home use.

A home steam "bath" is relatively simple to construct. It basically requires only these extra items: a prebuilt false floor for the bathtub, a long hose from the sink or a short hose attachment in the bathtub, a stool, and a large plastic sheet to create a "tent."

The false bottom should be made of a sturdy, nonsplintering material, and should have perforations for the steam to seep through. It should be elevated 4 inches. Place the false bottom in the tub. Place a stool on it. Attach a hose to the tub outlet or to a nearby sink. Create a plastic tent over the sides of the tub and your body. Only your head should be out. Open the hot-water faucet. The steam will emerge through the perforations. Place a cold compress on your forehead, and use a towel to close any gaps in the tent. Once the routine is established, it may be repeated several times a week provided that you don't get dizzy. The steam may be prepared somewhat in advance. Be careful not to burn yourself.

SAUNA

Therapeutic Uses

- Relieve fatigue
- Relieve arthritis

- Recover after exercise
- Relieve rheumatism
- Relieve skin problems (chronic eczema, psoriasis)
- Increase circulation
- Eliminate internal waste
- Help with menstrual disorders
- Increase perspiration
- Relieve joint pain

Many accident victims or arthritis patients find that the dry heat of the Finnish sauna helps them to function in a more normal manner. There is an intense but tolerable heat in the sauna room, and this causes profuse perspiration within a few minutes. The ideal way is to perspire, then take a tepid or a cool shower, and then plunge (if the sauna is at a gym) into a cold pool of water. The total effect of these three water activities creates a feeling of great cleanliness and exhilaration. The body soon develops the capacity to repeat this process frequently.

Control the tendency for headache or dizziness by applying a cold compress to the forehead.

Portable home saunas are commercially available.

TONIC TECHNIQUES

In increasing order of tonic effect:

1. Wet hand rub
2. Cold mitten friction massage
3. Alternate long hot and short cold sectional (Scots) shower
4. Cold towel rub
5. Pail pour
6. Salt rub before bath
7. Cold shower

The following cold showers should be preceded by a warm or hot shower. Start in only one section of the body, such as the feet or legs, and later add the spinal area or chest. The tonic effect is increased by the percussion of water.

- Wet sheet rub
- Dripping sheet rub

- Cold shower and cold bath
- Cold plunge

General Tonic: Use alternating long hot and short cold percussion showers directed to the legs, spine, and feet.

To Produce a Reaction in a Person Unaccustomed to Cold Application: Use a hot spray and then an alternate long hot and very short cold percussion shower directed to the spine and legs simultaneously.

Strengthening the Body

Cold water helps to restore strength and invigorate the body. When cold water is applied to only one section of the body at a time, it restores health, creates tone, overcomes energy blocks, and creates new circulation patterns.

Treading in Cold Water: Start with a 1-minute walk and work up to a 5-minute walk. Walk in water that is up to the knees. Cold-water treading influences the entire body: It strengthens the system; activates the kidneys, the bowels, and the bladder; facilitates breathing; and eliminates flatulence.

Simultaneous Arm and Footbath: This is a little tricky to arrange, but I've done it by standing in the bathtub and leaning over to the sink for the arm bath. Or you might use a container for the feet and a container on a table for the arm bath. Use cold water for both baths.

This bath strengthens the body. It is excellent during the recovery period after a long illness. It can be used by those with cold hand problems or for minor frostbite. Take the bath for 1 minute. Avoid chilling the body, because it negates the result.

Knee Showers: Warm the body in a bath or with a shower, and then direct a cold water shower to the knees at high pressure. This is a very powerful treatment and should not be used for more than 3 or 4 days. However, should you wish to continue this treatment, follow this sequence: Direct the jet spray first to the knees, then to the arms, then to the upper body.

To Toughen the Body

I love the cold-water ankle splash. It's a great wakeup routine, and it is a remarkable sleep aid if used just before going to bed. And of course cold-water therapy of any kind helps you to mobilize your immune system as well as adapt your body to cold temperatures.

It takes time to get used to this intrepid therapy, so I suggest you start off with a few seconds' splash and gradually increase the time as you become more tolerant of the cold. You'll not only feel better and sleep better, since this therapy greatly increases circulation, but as the days and weeks of winter go on, the cold weather should bother you less and less.

If you think the cold ankle splashes take a lot of courage, can you imagine dousing yourself outdoors with ice-cold water in the wintertime? On a visit to Japan, at 5:30 each morning I watched the neighbors, dressed only in *fundoshi*, first dousing themselves with pails of cold water, then exuberantly scrubbing themselves with a stiff brush. These stalwart aikido practitioners told me of others who purified and hardened themselves under a waterfall.

PERSPIRATION INDUCTION

The human body has a network of 2 million sweat glands and about 6 miles of ducts on the skin. During illness, the ducts do not work as well as they should and need stimulation. This is easily accomplished without drugs by using the simple techniques of water therapy. Water therapy helps to rebalance and normalize body health by rushing unneeded toxins and surplus waste materials out of the body in the form of perspiration. This process also stimulates the kidneys so that they function better, relieves internal congestion, decreases edema, and helps to prepare even the weakest patient for possible cold-water therapy.

When only the edema or restricted blood flow remains, direct alternate hot and cold percussion showers to the area.

Take rosemary baths to increase circulation.

Water Treatments to Induce Perspiration

- Sunbathing
- Turkish or Russian steamroom bath
- Sauna

- Full hot bath (herbs optional)
- Dry pack
- Cold damp (or dripping wet) sheet compress—partial or full
- Hot shower
- Hot footbath, hot leg bath
- Hot shallow sit bath
- Hot moist application to spine
- Hot blanket pack—partial or full
- Drinking hot water
- Heat edema
- Steam tent or vaporizer

Hot Herb Baths, Steam Rooms, Saunas, Hot Tubs

Sweating it out is good for you. It is a natural cure. It is amazing how you can relieve headaches and nausea and a general feeling of malaise by simply eliminating toxins through the 2 million sweat glands of the skin. Exercisers like to use saunas and steam rooms because the steam flushes out lactic acid, the cause of stiff muscles and much normal fatigue. Ninety-eight percent of the sweat is water, but the rest is full of toxins such as salt, heavy metals, nicotine, and other chemicals found in the environment.

Provide a detoxifying sweat bath at home. Read the information on hayflower, Epsom salts, or fennel seed. You can also drink peppermint tea or ginger tea to induce excretion through the skin.

What is the story on public saunas and steam rooms?

The results of a survey conducted by Dr. Edward Press, professor emeritus at Oregon Health Sciences University School of Medicine and former Oregon state public health officer, show that deaths from becoming overheated in saunas and from drowning in hot tubs can and do occur. People may pass out and cannot summon help, or they develop abnormal heart rhythms and go into cardiac arrest.

Dr. Press cautions that the air temperature in a sauna should not exceed 176°F (80°C), nor should the water in a whirlpool exceed 104°F (40°C). According to Dr. Press, those with hypertension and other cardiac conditions and those drinking alcohol or sniffing cocaine are at high risk. Patients with diabetes and epilepsy are particularly at risk, and Press advises them not to spend more than five minutes in a spa or a sauna.

How long should a session in a sauna, steam room, or hot tub last? That depends on the person and his or her tolerance to heat. Some people stay in a long time, others like to leave as soon as they start to perspire. Europeans who are knowledgeable about water therapy end "sweats" with cold dunks or cool showers. If you prefer to take a warm shower, at least end the shower with cool to moderately cold water.

The precautions: Don't take a hot steamy bath or enter a sauna, steam room, or hot tub for at least one hour after eating. The reason for this limitation is that you need your blood to be circulating near the skin, not in your digestive system. To prevent dehydration, drink a significant amount of water. Try to replace the potassium lost to perspiration by eating a banana or an orange. Never stay in the sauna or steam room if you feel the slightest discomfort. If you have hypertension or heart trouble, keep out of the sauna, steam room, or whirlpool hot tub. Recent studies have shown that while heat stress from a sauna generally won't cause blood pressure changes in nonhypertensive people, hypertensives on medication may experience a significant drop in blood pressure, which may lead to dizziness or fainting. This leads to a faster heartbeat and in some cases to a heart attack.

Can you get genital herpes in a steam room or hot tub or on the benches of a sauna? Researchers failed to find live herpes virus in the hot tubs, but they were able to demonstrate that live herpes virus can survive on tile and plastic surfaces in moist, warm areas. I interviewed a world-famous dermatologist, a specialist in sexually transmitted diseases, who told me that as a result of her work she would never go into a public hot tub. "There are too many possibilities for bacterial growth in that intense heat," she confided. A public hot tub that is not scrupulously clean can also spread such bacterial infections as boils and conjunctivitis.

Researchers have also investigated dermatitis outbreaks from public hot tub whirlpools. According to R. A. Breitenbach of the Department of Academic Family Medicine, Wayne State University School of Medicine, Detroit, low disinfectant levels and inadequate monitoring are clearly a public health concern. He cautions physicians to be on the alert for well-demarcated rashes that may be associated with improperly maintained whirlpools.

In 1989 the medical journal *The Lancet* reported on an outbreak of Legionnaires' disease, a powerful and sometimes fatal form of pneumonia, in 187 people who had visited a hotel and leisure complex in a village on the west coast of Scotland. The outbreak was traced to the whirlpool spa.

CLAY

*K*eep a pound or two of neutral white or gray clay on hand (ceramic marmalade jugs are useful) for a wide variety of healing actions to alleviate diarrhea, burns, neuritis attacks, swellings, bruises, and some chronic pain. Clay can be used alone or mixed with an herbal oil, or an assortment of herbs for nerve inflammation problems. Clay water and herbal infusions, and heated leaves of cabbage or raw, grated potato are ideal rotation partners in reducing resistant skin swellings, even minor topical growths, and in lessening some arthritic pain.

APPLYING CLAY POULTICES

Clay can be added to an herbal oil, a strained herbal infusion or decoction, or pure water. Prepare a thin paste and apply the paste directly to the skin, or preferably, because it dries and flakes, on a clean white cloth or wide piece of gauze, which can be lifted intact from the problem area. To prevent the clay "peeling," cover the application with thin cloth strips, or loosely with an elastic bandage such as used for sports injuries. Or attach long Velcro straps to bind poultices. The straps are available in some rehabilitation specialty shops.

CHRONIC ARTHRITIC PAIN

For arthritic pain, combine clay and castor oil to make a healing poultice. Since clay soothes but does not bring circulation to the skin surface, interchange the clay and castor oil poultice with large heated cabbage leaf poultices. Cabbage draws out toxins (for this reason, it can be used to draw out pus from wounds, too). To create internal and surface circulation and heat, combine clay paste and tiny amounts of such counterirritant herbs as eucalyptus oil or juniper needle oil. An easy way to produce similar external heat is to combine clay and small quantities of Tiger Balm, an ointment containing five counterirritant herbs. Apply all of these in overnight poultices.

NERVE INFLAMMATION (NEURITIS)

Neuritis pain is insidious. Heat applications help. Do not use heating pads because of the danger of electromagnetic rays from these pads. Instead, use a combination of hot water compresses, hot water bottle applications, and/or heated herbal compresses. If these don't work, combine clay and a heated herbal oil to produce a thin, gummy paste. The two healing oils that are most effective are castor oil or St. John's wort oil. In a pinch you can use heated olive oil. The oil has four actions here: It provides its own healing power; makes the area feel warm; keeps the clay supple; and in the right combination prevents the clay from drying and flaking. Reinforce the heating action by initially applying a hot water bottle over the poultice. After the hot water bottle cools down, discard it, but keep the poultice on as long as you can, preferably overnight. This can be repeated as often as needed.

The herb lemon balm is also effective for neuritis pain. Make the lemon balm into a strong tea, strain, and add as a source of liquid to the clay for a thin poultice application. Comfrey liquid can be added to clay poultices to relieve pressure and nerve damage pain. If only ointment of comfrey is available, alternate gentle topical applications of the ointment with clay poultices, or any of the clay plus herb poultices.

DIARRHEA

Clay pellets or clay diluted in a glass of water are helpful in treating most kinds of diarrhea. Do not take any but the purest clay internally. Add any quieting herbal infusion (tea) to the clay water. Since pure Coca-Cola syrup (or Classic Coke) is especially useful in diarrhea, you can combine a mashed pellet of clay in pure water plus a dollop of Coke syrup. Activated charcoal tablets are also valuable for diarrhea. Like the clay, such tablets absorb the internal toxins causing the diarrhea attack.

BURNS

The first, most successful remedy for minor burns is ice-water application. But sometimes even when the ice water cleanses the charred area (it becomes clean and white), there is still residual pain that causes throbbing. Add a thin "mask" of clay over the newly healed burn to further heal and shield the area from the air. This absence of air soothes the pain and influences healing. Since the clay dries and sheds, wind a light layer of gauze over the clay. If the pain persists, apply a fresh dose of wet clay to keep out the air.

SWELLINGS AND SMALL GROWTHS

Herbs and clays have been used for thousands of years to diminish swellings and some growths. Some success has been reported with the use of castor oil poultices, alone or in combination with clay paste poultices. Several herbs are said to be effective in reducing bumps, swellings, and new growths. Add these herbs to clay poultices: strained horsetail infusion (tea), an infusion of marigold (calendula) tea, strained oak bark decoction (simmered "soup" of bark), or blended ground-up bran plus a little water.

Heated organic cabbage leaf poultices can be alternated with the various clay poultices. To lessen possible skin reactions, such as blisters on sensitive skin, before applying the heated and softened cabbage leaf, first pat on a thin layer of oil. Some people may have an initial period of mild pain in response to the powerful, detoxifying cabbage application. The pain will subside.

Raw, grated organic potato poultices can also be used alternately with clay poultices on a variety of bruises, inflammations, slow-healing wounds, and wounds with pus discharges. Combine the grated potato with milk and apply directly to the skin, or use it as a poultice encased in gauze or clean cloth. Depending on one's reaction to cold and heat, potato poultices can be used warm or cold.

Very resistant swellings often respond to a rotation series of poultices of clay and warm oil, cabbage, and then potato. These three actions and sequences can be repeated.

part 3
Water Healing for Common Ailments

ABSCESS

An abscess is a localized collection of pus. An acute abscess can produce fever and a painful local inflammation.

Water Therapy

Internal: In general, keep the bowels clear. Each morning upon arising drink 1 to 2 glasses of cold water. For an attack of an abscess (or boil), purify the body for three days with a glass of beet, carrot, or mixed greens juice. If the abscess is internal, cleanse the body every half-hour with hot chamomile tea gargles and drinks.

For a mouth abscess, rinse out the mouth as often as possible. Alternate hot chamomile tea gargles and drinks with this mouth-friendly, antiseptic herbal combination: Combine 3 to 4 drops tincture of myrrh with 4 drops of goldenseal tincture (or a pinch of goldenseal powder) in a glass of water. Rinse through the mouth several times a day.

External (Poultices): Goldenseal is toxic to the bacteria in abscesses and boils. It decreases inflammation even while it jolts and sustains the immune system. Moisten several tablespoons of goldenseal powder. Place on a clean cloth and fold into a tiny cloth envelope. Place on the abscess.

Silica 6x in either tissue salt or homeopathic form will help the abscess to ripen and discharge. Dissolve one or two silica 6x pills in half a glass of water. Dip a disposable square cloth in the hot water, wring out, and apply while warm to the abscess.

General Therapy

Fight the internal infection in one or all of these three ways.

1. Use garlic in food or take 2 to 3 deodorized garlic capsules as a safe and strong antibactericide.
2. Add the two infection-fighter vitamins, vitamin C (as ascorbic acid powder or in ester form) and vitamin A (in emulsion form) to fight the internal infection. Holistic physicians use high doses of these vitamins to clear internal infections. *Vitamin C:* 2,000 mg to 3,000 mg (depending on bowel tolerance) spaced out during the day. *Vitamin A:* Fresh carrot juice contains about 18,000 IU of vitamin A per glass. Try 1½ glasses, or start with a 25,000 IU dose of tablets for a few days. During an emergency such as this, holistic physicians work up to 50,000 IU and higher. In addition, take 50 mg of a B complex vitamin and 30 mg zinc to protect against future attacks; 400 IU of vitamin E; 1 tablespoon of liquid chlorophyll twice a day to purify the system; and 50 mg coenzyme Q10 each day to increase oxygen and enhance the immune system.
3. Cell salts: Dissolve 5 tablets of ferrum phos. 6x under the tongue at the first indication of an oncoming abscess or boil. Continue this therapy until the inflammation abates.

ACNE

Water Therapy

Blackhead Extractor: You will need a kettle of boiling water, several very soft washcloths, Epsom salts, white iodine tincture, and white tissues. Boil 2 cups of water in a nonaluminum pot and drop in 1 tablespoon of Epsom salts and

3 drops of white iodine. Keep it hot on a stove or an electric hot tray. Soak several clean, soft washcloths in the steaming hot water. Open the pores of the face with a chamomile steam facial. When the pores are open, take one of the soaking washcloths and apply it, as hot as possible, on the first embedded blackhead. Press the blackhead out with a tissue. The blackhead should pop out. After the blackhead is extracted, close the pore with cold water and a splash of astringent witch hazel. Continue with the hot Epsom salt and white iodine treatment, one blackhead at a time.

General Therapy

Tea tree oil is an excellent herbal antibacterial aid. Combine 4 drops of the oil with 4 tablespoons of witch hazel (purchase at drugstore). Dip a cotton swab into the preparation and apply to pimples. Avoid contamination by using one swab for each pimple.

There are 38 Bach flower remedies designed to combat mood fluctuations. If you have feelings of discomfort, "uncleanliness," or embarrassment about the acne outbreak, 4 drops of crabapple remedy under the tongue or in half a glass of water chases these feelings away.

Eliminate junk food, exercise regularly (this increases internal circulation and helps to eliminate toxins), walk in the sunshine for a few minutes each day, breathe in fresh air in a conscious manner. Meditate to overcome stress. If you take antibiotics, absolutely take yogurt-rich acidophilus or acidophilus capsules to counter a potential yeast infection.

There are several excellent sulphur-rich preparations for cleansing the skin, such as Akne-Zyme (but avoid it before and during pregnancy) and Derma-Klear Akne Treatment Cleanser (and cream).

ARTHRITIS

Water Therapy

Drink water—lots of it. The synovial fluid, which lubricates the joints, consists primarily of water. Although arthritis is a disease of the entire system and responds to a wide variety of coordinated therapies, one theory postulates that arthritis is caused by dehydration in which a lack of essential synovial fluid can later precipitate chronic arthritis.

Use ice packs on any inflamed joint. Purchase several large, soft gel "cold packs" and keep them in the freezer. Use them as needed during the day. To improve a night's sleep, wind one around an inflamed joint with an elastic or Velcro bandage for about 10 to 15 minutes. Amazing what a little icing can do.

In addition to rapid/short cold applications, arthritis patients can find relief in moist heat applications. This includes a fast hot needle shower to get the day started, which can be further stimulated if alternate hot and cold sprays are applied. Use long bursts of hot and short bursts of cold, and end on the cold. Even better for relaxing stiff muscles is the long and leisurely hot bath. Dribble in some colder water at the end to awaken the body. This same hot bath, possibly with pine, melissa, or other oils, 1 hour before bedtime, will ensure a rapid start to profound sleep. Whenever possible massage the body with almond, calendula (marigold), or peanut oil.

A double cold-water heating compress will relieve pain by sending heat to an inflamed area from within the system. This procedure should work within 10 minutes. If it doesn't, take it off. It can be used freely unless you are weak, feeble, or immunocompromised. Dip a long strip of cotton cloth into cold water. Wring it out. Wrap it around the inflamed joint and close it with a safety pin. Immediately cover the wet compress with a wool strip (an old, soft wool scarf is perfect). Fasten with a safety pin so that no air can penetrate to the cold compress. The body has a wisdom of its own and immediately sends fresh blood to the cold area to warm it up. The area soon feels cozy and warm. The compress can be left on for a half-hour or more.

Castor oil packs are exceptionally healing and may be used on a long-term basis, about one half-hour at a time. Fold a flannel (preferred) or cotton cloth into a square a little larger than the joint that needs healing. Drizzle on a layer of castor oil (see Resources) and apply the oiled side to the affected joint. Cover the pack with a larger piece of plastic and attach the pack and plastic cover firmly with an elastic bandage or a long Velcro strap. When finished, the oiled cloths can be saved in a plastic bag for future applications.

Try these poultices over a series of three days. On the first day, apply a poultice of pulped cabbage leaves; on the second day, apply a poultice of neutral clay; and on the third day, apply a poultice of soft white cheese. Another excellent poultice for arthritic pains can be prepared with corn or millet porridge, both of which are thought to increase circulation. Apply the poultice as hot as you can tolerate it. Another great remedy for arthritis is a hot pack (poultice) of hayseed applied to the area of joint pain.

Hot wax will ease the pain. Until recently such hot wax treatments were only available at physiotherapists and pain treatment specialists, but the paraffin and an electric machine are now available by mail. (See Resources.) Heat the wax and place the arthritic hand, finger, or foot into the hot wax. As soon as a film of wax settles over the painful site, withdraw it from the heat. Enjoy the effect of the hot paraffin. Peel off the wax when the heat subsides and return the wax to the electric tub. It can be used again and again.

Drinking Water: Drink 8 glasses of pure water each day to flush the system of impurities and to hydrate the joints. Distilled water is preferred by many alternative and complementary practitioners, who believe this type of water binds mineral salts and vegetable acids, which help to eliminate waste products through the kidneys.

Baths: Herbal baths are highly effective in treating rheumatic conditions. To prepare a bath that will stimulate circulation, crush a handful of dried calamus root and a handful of dried thyme leaves. Fold into cheesecloth (tie with a rubberband) or place in a large stainless steel container. Drop into a full tub of moderately hot water.

Perspiration: Baths are also useful in eliminating toxins through the skin. To promote perspiration use neutral (slightly less than body temperature, 95°F) baths. A cup of Epsom salts in slightly warmer or even hot water will promote profuse perspiration. If one is robust, these baths can be taken about once a week or less. Such baths are remarkable in their action, but deplete the store of energy. Never go outside immediately after such a bath, but rather take the bath before a nap or bedtime.

Three other herbs create only moderate perspiration but are nevertheless considered exceptionally detoxifying. Add several drops of a tincture, or a handful of dried hayflowers, oatstraw, or bruised fennel seeds (encased in cheesecloth) to the bathwater once or twice a month.

Colon Irrigation: To increase circulation.

ASTHMA

Asthma attacks are terrifying to both the sufferer and his or her family, and anxiety about an attack can aggravate another one.

There are several causes. One type of attack is initiated by sensitivity to pollen, molds, animal danders, lint, or insecticide. Another is caused by an infection in the nose, sinus, or lower lungs, and such attacks can be set off by changes in temperature, humidity, or exposure to chemical, paint, or wax fumes. Others are caused by exhaustion, changes in endocrine balance during puberty, menstruation, pregnancy, and menopause. Many attacks are triggered by emotional stress.

Asthma sufferers should avoid the allergens they are sensitive to, and try not to become fatigued.

Water Therapy

Water therapy has the unique ability to shift blood from a more congested area of the body to a less congested part. It can be utilized in the case of an asthma attack to lessen chest pain and spasms. Since there are a variety of possible approaches, experiment with all of them to see which helps you in controlling an attack.

In an emergency, use one or all of the following quick-acting techniques. Have one or more of the following items ready to use: a cold pack or ice in the freezer; English mustard powder for a footbath (found on grocery shelves or at pharmacies); coffee in the freezer; apple cider vinegar; an enema bag (drugstore); a steam inhaler or ways of improvising steam; and one or several herbs ready for the steam inhalation.

As a preventive, make sure to drink enough water each day. One theory suggests that asthma may be a result of dehydration. It seems that if the body does not maintain enough water for necessary functioning, it begins to conserve water, including releasing histamines into the lungs, which in turn constricts the bronchioles to prevent water loss, triggering the symptoms of asthma.

Apply an ice bag to the back of the head.

Place the feet in a hot footbath. Provide extra zing with a tablespoon of dried mustard powder.

Immerse the hands in hot water for a few seconds or longer.

At the onset of an attack consider drinking 1 to 3 cups of coffee. Coffee contains theophylline, a common substance in asthma medications.

The late Swiss master-herbalist Johann Kunzle used this hot cider arm compress as a blood diversion technique to alleviate an acute asthma attack: Bring to a boil several cups of slightly fermented old cider or apple cider vinegar. Take off the heat and soak several clean dishtowels in the liquid. As soon as you can tolerate the heat, wring out one of the towels and wrap it around the left arm. As soon as the cloth loses heat, apply another hot cloth to the right arm. Apply and alternate the hot compresses until the chest pain subsides.

The late Bavarian master-herbalist Sebastian Kneipp used another hot apple cider vinegar technique to divert blood flow to relieve pressure on the chest. He advised his asthma patients to apply a hot vinegar compress to the stomach, saying, "As soon as artificial warmth is generated in the stomach, it spreads to the chest and diverts the blood downwards, making the pain more bearable and eventually removing it." To make this compress, heat 2 cups of apple cider vinegar and soak several flannel or cotton cloths in the liquid. Wring out one cloth and apply it directly and gently to the stomach. Kneipp also advised this hot enema for asthma-induced intestinal or kidney spasms: Fill the enema bag with warm to hot water from the tap. Test the heat of the water first on the hand, then internally. If the water is too hot, add some cooler water. Kneipp's patients used this enema treatment every half-hour until the spasms stopped.

Steam inhalation is a direct water therapy. It is useful with asthma to clear the system and dissolve chest congestion. Such a steam inhalation may be used as a preventive measure once a week during stable periods, or every other day during periods of asthma attacks. In an emergency, a hot bathroom shower (with the door closed) can create a steamy room. Otherwise use a store-bought steam inhaler (see Resources), or improvise a steam-vapor "tent." Boil water in a large pot, take it off the stove, and place it on a safe kitchen table. Create a tent-like effect with a large towel and sit under the tent with eyes closed for about 10 minutes. If possible, add any of these healing herbs to the boiling water: leaves of sage or nettle; flowers of linden, elder, or yarrow.

General Therapy

Tongue Hardening: Dr. William Fitzgerald, the late ear, nose, and throat specialist who invented Zone Therapy, had two preventive tips for his asthma patients:

1. Have the teeth checked often.
2. Ward off future coughing fits by "hardening" the tongue: Lightly clench it between the teeth for 3 to 4 minutes a day.

Breathing Exercise: A helpful breathing exercise is to sit with your elbows and hands on your knees. The position relieves breathlessness by stretching the diaphragm upward.

Tips for Exercise–Induced Asthma: Exercise sometimes induces an asthma attack when the air is cold and dry. These two approaches have been found helpful: Breathe through pursed lips—this raises internal air pressure in the chest passage. Wear a surgical mask during exercise. The mask allows you to breathe your own moist air rather than breathing outside cold air, which can act as an irritant.

BACK (LOWER BACK PROBLEMS)

Water Therapy

Apply either a frozen bandage or an ice pack to the painful area. If you don't have an ice pack, a bag of frozen peas works well. Frozen bandages must be prepared in advance and stored in the freezer. (See section on "Ice" in Part 2 for directions.) If you have an herbal or homeopathic liniment, rub it on the body before applying the ice pack. I've had great luck with homeopathic arnica ointment. Another good bet is the over-the-counter herbal ointment Tiger Balm, which contains five circulation-inducing herbs. I prefer the white ointment to the red because it doesn't stain clothes. Other good ointments are Olbas ointment or anything containing eucalyptus or wintergreen.

Dehydration greatly influences muscle fatigue and acid buildup in the muscles. If your back hurts, drink two glasses of water immediately. Another reason to drink water is to overcome and prevent constipation, a hidden cause of many chronic back pain attacks.

Stand under a shower and alternate both hot and cold sprays to the area of back pain. Always end with a cool spray. If it isn't possible to take a shower, alternate hot and cold compresses to the painful area.

Sit in a hot hip (sitz) bath for 10 minutes. Prevent chills by covering the upper torso with a towel. To heal and tranquilize the entire body, take a neutral-temperature bath. During the bath, promote additional circulation with friction rubs. Use either a dry bath brush, a large sponge, or a rough washcloth or loofah.

BAD BREATH

Water Therapy

Bad breath can be caused by many factors, including poor mouth hygiene and constipation. Water therapy is essential for proper mouth hygiene.

Swish water through the mouth immediately after eating.

Avoid constipation by drinking 2 glasses of cold water upon waking.

Drink no less than 8 glasses of clear water a day to encourage saliva to wash away food deposits and mouth bacteria.

Humidify the bedroom area with a small humidifier (it should be cleaned every night) or by a placing fresh pot of water in the bedroom every evening.

Concoct a home mouthwash by combining 1 teaspoon of vodka per cup to any of the following steeped and strained herbal teas: bruised cloves, fennel seeds, aniseed, dill seeds, cardamom seeds, cinnamon, peppermint, rosemary, sage, or thyme. Store in the refrigerator.

General Therapy

Avoid eating smelly foods. One of the best old-fashioned remedies to cleanse the system and filter out smelly or gassy foods is an occasional tablet of activated charcoal. These activated charcoal tablets are available in pharmacies and health food stores. Also add an occasional acidophilus capsule to your diet, eat several green vegetables each day, and/or add liquid chlorophyll or tablets to your daily diet (take between meals). Chew raw carrots and apples to cleanse the mouth between frequent brushing and flossing.

BEDWETTING

Water Therapy

There are several preventive water therapy measures for bedwetting. The early German and Austrian hydrotherapists all used external cold-water therapies to strengthen the body.

For adults, Kneipp successfully used 3- to 4-minute sessions of cold-water treading (standing and/or walking in water) up to the calves. Within one week all patients showed remarkable results. Continue this cold-water treading to maintain vitality and body tone. End each session with either a brief cold arm bath or a friction rub with a washcloth.

For children, use cold water in this way: Briefly dip toddlers (up to four years) in cold water. Start with a 1-second dip, and as tolerance to the cold builds up, gradually increase the dips up to 3 seconds. Children older than four years can hold onto a rail or a parent while they march for several seconds in cold water up to their calves. The tolerance to the cold is soon built up and the water should feel pleasant. The room must be free of drafts, and children should be dried as soon as each procedure ends. If the child is resistant to walking in the cold water, try brief cold-water friction rubs with a washcloth on the feet up to the calves. On occasion, warm water compresses can be used. To stimulate the blood circulation of the urinary organs, place a warm, moist hayflower compress on the lower part of the abdomen every day.

Sometimes an enema is needed to stimulate and cleanse the area. Jethro Kloss, an eminent nineteenth-century naturopath, felt a clogged colon could be a cause of some bedwetting problems. Therefore, if a child tends to be constipated, utilize a gentle bulb syringe enema to rid the colon of putrefied matter. If an enema is out of the question, try a gentle herbal laxative such as a quarter to a half tablet of Inner Clean. (Adults can take one tablet.)

Dr. Rudolf Fritz Weiss, the German physician and botanical researcher, tells us that St. John's wort (*Hypericum perforatum*) "acts via the nervous system in the treatment of bedwetting. St. John's wort, which has just been rediscovered by the entire world as an effective antidepressant, has also been judged to be highly productive in clinical trials of enuresis (bedwetting)." Other herbs that are successful for bedwetting are sweet marjoram tea; 20 drops of gentian tincture in a glass of water at midday and in the evening; or chamomile or linden tea to relax a tense child.

In addition, on occasion, before bedtime, take a 10-minute hot shallow (sitz) bath followed by a few seconds cold sitz bath. Dry the body and go to bed immediately.

General Therapy

In general, urinate as often as possible after supper, particularly one hour before bedtime, and also restrict fluid intake after supper. It is helpful to add a multiple vitamin to the diet as well as a B-complex supplement, and since bedwetters are often deficient in B_2 (riboflavin) and pantothenic acid, add these Bs in addition. Sometimes bedwetting occurs because of a slight misalignment of the spine. For this reason, most bedwetting children respond to a gentle buttock massage, and both children and adults show results from chiropractic and/or osteopathic adjustments.

BODY ODOR

Water Therapy

Water may be used in four distinct ways as an essential therapy for body odor.

Drinking Water: Drinking at least 2 quarts of water daily hydrates the cells, cleanses the digestive system, and stimulates the kidneys to excrete clear urine. This amount of water flushes the kidneys and helps to overcome a possible minor kidney malfunction. Such a breakdown can affect body odor because it can force toxins that normally go out through the kidneys to emerge through the skin. Fennel tea is highly purifying and may be added to drinking water any time of the day.

Baths: Steeping the body in a bath changes the pH of the skin and increases elimination of toxins through cleansing and sweating. Reestablish the proper pH of the skin by splashing and sponging the body with apple cider vinegar and adding 1 to 2 cups of apple cider vinegar to the bath. Use apple cider vinegar as a deodorant under the armpits. These herbs also function as useful deodorants: fennel, chamomile, rosemary, sage, red clover, thyme, and cinnamon.

Sweating: Epsom salts (magnesium sulphate) in a bath causes profuse sweating. Add about 1 cup to hot water and soak for 10 to 15 minutes. The bath is exceedingly sedating and depleting, so take it just before bedtime. A hayflower extract bath is also exceptionally detoxifying. Once a week take a sauna or steam bath to sweat out internal toxins. Epsom salt baths, saunas, and steam rooms should not be taken by pregnant women and those with heart or circulation problems.

Internal Streams of Water: Cleanse hardened internal waste material with a series of warm-water enemas.

General Therapy

Chew 2 chlorophyll plant tablets with each meal. Because some body odor seems to occur because of a slight zinc deficiency, take a good multi-mineral-vitamin with the normal RDA of zinc.

BURSITIS

Water Therapy

Apply ice during acute attack periods to diminish the pain and decrease the swelling. Switch to heat treatments after two days. Use any of these hot water treatments: a hot spray shower, alternate long hot and short snappy cold spray showers, a hot pack compress on the area of the pain, or general hot baths.

General Therapy

Internal: Ingest 4 tablets of homeopathic arnica 6x for the pain.

External: Apply arnica 6x homeopathic ointment to control the pain or apply a cayenne pepper (capsicum) ointment to the area of the pain. This ointment, which is available over the counter in pharmacies, takes between ten days to two weeks to start working. Massage with castor oil or apply castor oil packs to the area. If the area is misaligned, a chiropractor or an osteopath can restore mobility and range of motion. However, there are times when an adjustment can aggravate bursitis, so discuss the problem in advance. A series of TENS (transcutaneous electrical neural stimulator) applications will usually reduce the pain.

CANKER SORES

Water Therapy

Numb the pain by stroking an ice cube on the sore.

To promote healing, stimulate circulation, and soothe pain, rinse the mouth several times a day with warm salt water. Or rinse the mouth with the following strong herbal teas: red raspberry leaf, burdock, sage, or red clover.

Rinse with goldenseal powder combined with drops of myrrh tincture. This takes the pain away immediately and heals the area quickly.

General Therapy

Acidophilus culture is a preventive treatment for patients with recurring canker sores. Take in capsule form or with a yogurt that contains acidophilus. Dr. J. B. Chapman, in *Biochemistry: Twelve Biochemic Remedies*, believes that canker sores occur both in children and adults because of a mineral deficiency of Kali mur., and says it "is the chief and generally, the only remedy required." Kali mur. comes in cell salt (tissue salt) and homeopathic form. The adult dose is 5 tablets under the tongue. Give 2 tablets to a child. Repeat several times a day if necessary.

CARPAL TUNNEL SYNDROME

Carpal tunnel syndrome repair is now the second most frequent surgical procedure in America as a result of the long hours we spend at computer keyboards with our hands and elbows in unnatural and uncomfortable positions.

Water Therapy

Dip the hands in extremely hot water as often as possible. Fifteen years or so ago, I had a chronic case of carpal tunnel syndrome, which began when I worked on a keyboard and was aggravated by carrying shopping bags loaded with food on a long train trip. Each night I awakened with the pain and pins and needles in my hands, and I used hot water immersion to relieve the pain.

General Therapy

My managed care physician insisted on an operation. When I told him I wanted to find an alternative, he said, "Don't come back to me when your hand falls off!" I was shocked by his dire prediction, but luckily I found an alternative treatment. A writing colleague, Ruth Winter, told me that her husband (the eminent neurosurgeon Arthur Winter) had been experimenting with electrical pulsating pain control for his surgery patients. Arthur believed the same apparatus, a TENS (transcutaneous electrical neural stimulator) machine might cure my carpal tunnel problems. Although not everyone responds to electrical stimulation, he was right on target in my case. He placed one pad on the fleshy part of the thumb and the second pad on the palm right under the pinky and ring fingers. After the initial treatment, the pain disappeared for five days, but then returned. I needed a series of seven weekly visits for the pain to disappear. Because I was such a chronic and old case, I believe it may have taken me longer than a new case. These days physiotherapists all use one or another version of the TENS machine to alleviate pain—so go for treatments, or rent a machine for your own treatments.

CHRONIC FATIGUE SYNDROME

Water Therapy

Chronic fatigue syndrome is a complicated health problem that requires a multi-disciplinary approach, only one part of which is water therapy, which helps to relax, cleanse, and purify the body and to stimulate lassitude.

Drink 8 or more glasses of water every day to cleanse and purify the system. Also drink these healing liquids: fresh carrot juice, or carrot combined with celery, beet, or sour apple.

To stimulate the system and to encourage detoxification, dry-brush the body on arising and before taking a shower or bath.

Each day when tired, splash some apple cider vinegar on the chest, shoulders, and upper arms. The apple cider vinegar restores the skin to its normal pH and helps to overcome normal fatigue.

Restore circulation and achieve a fresh feeling of well-being with a coarse salt rub while in the bath. Coarse salt, such as Kosher salt, can be found in the supermarket. Use between a handful to a half-pound in the bath to refresh the body, and apply slightly diluted as a body rub on the shoulders, torso, arms, thighs, and knees. This can be done several times a week to energize and restore the body.

As frequently as needed, take alternate hot and brief cold showers (end in cold) to exhilarate and stimulate the body. Avoid them if you are pregnant or have heart or circulatory problems.

To encourage easy sleep, relax in a warm to hot bath each day one hour before bedtime.

If there are headaches or any other upper body congestion, try occasional brief hot footbaths. Avoid them if you have any circulatory problems or diabetes.

General Therapy

Acupuncture can help with fatigue, possible short-term memory loss, depression, joint and muscle pain, devitalized sleep problems, concentration, and other problems. Mild gradual exercise provides several recovery essentials. In addition to helping to overcome depression, it helps to rid the body of toxins and free radicals, which deplete the immune system. Exercise will also overcome lassitude and provide a sense of new and needed energy. Massage treatments, chiropractic adjustments to stimulate circulation and restore the spine to its optimum function, yoga classes to overcome shallow breathing, and support groups are all very helpful.

COLDS

Water Therapy

Wash your hands with soap, often! Hand washing is deadly to a cold. Whether you are staggering from a big one or wrestling with a sniffle, germs are spread via the fingers. Avoid touching your eyes and nose, and refrain from sharing obvious germ-carrying objects like drinking glasses and phones, computer keyboards and pencils. Dispose of tissues, paper towels, and drinking containers promptly.

Drink copious amounts of water. Start early in the morning and reach for a glass of water in place of soda, coffee, or tea. Drink hot lemonade and honey, herbal teas, and clear broth throughout the day.

Every morning, wash your nose by sluicing both nostrils with a saline solution (salt water) and drying with a tissue. This is a key, and underemployed, way to cut off a cold.

Massage your big toe with ice.

To help the body detoxify and perspire, and shed the oncoming or active cold, take a hot bath with a hayflower bath extract (Biokosma), or a detoxifying Epsom salts bath. (Avoid this last one if you are pregnant or have heart or circulation problems.) Get right into bed and perspire away.

If you are seriously stuffed up, a hot footbath (especially with 1 tablespoon of mustard seed powder) can temporarily draw the congestion to the feet and away from the head.

Another way to release stuffiness is to draw congestion away from the head with the cold stocking application. Wet knee-high cotton stockings. Wring out the water and put them on your feet. Immediately pull on long wool stockings over the wet cotton ones. The body should send heat to the area immediately and the feet will warm up and draw the congestion away from the nose. Do not do this if you are feeble, very old, or very young. If the feet don't warm up quickly, discard the application.

Sometimes a neutral-temperature enema is necessary to cleanse the whole system and abort a cold.

Wash your hair daily, taking care to vigorously massage the entire head. Touching vital head trigger points jumpstarts the healing process. Dry your hair immediately to avoid a chill.

Humidify the bedroom. A hot steam humidifier (see Resources) helps to clear clogged nasal passages.

Once in bed, drink ginger tea or a ginger toddy (ginger in whisky), peppermint tea with ginger slices, or drink Jamaican ginger ale (Reeds), which is a lot like home-brewed ginger ale.

General Therapy

Want to stop drizzling from the nose almost instantly? I am a long-term devotee of Dr. William Fitzgerald's rubber band Zone Therapy. For a cold, wind a wide rubber band around the knuckle of one thumb at a time.

Start with the thumb on the side of the nostril with the strongest "drip." As Fitzgerald suggested, continue to wear the restricting rubber band until the area not only looks purple (that's OK), but starts to hurt. It works like a personalized form of pressure acupuncture. Yes, you can use it in the bath!

To abort a cold before it takes hold, try any anti-cold homeopathic tablet(s). I often use Boiron's combination called Cold Calm. Increase your immune function with extra vitamin C and echinacea. Suck zinc lozenges to combat the major loss of zinc that occurs with every infection. Purify the system by ingesting an activated charcoal tablet. Don't overtire yourself. Rest often. Walk in the fresh air whenever possible. Practice deep breathing to cleanse your lungs and tone your respiratory system. Sleep in a well-ventilated, humidified room.

COLD SORES

Water Therapy

Immediately massage the tingling area with an ice cube. Repeat every half-hour. The ice massage may prevent the cold sore from emerging.

Alternate the ice massage with continuous 3 hour hot saltwater compresses. Keep hot water on a stove or on an electric tray. Soak several cloths in the hot water. Withdraw one cloth at a time, wring out, and apply fairly hot to the tingling area. Replace the cloth as it cools. Swab the area with brandy every hour or so.

Drink at least 8 glasses of water each day.

General Therapy

Take preventive doses of 500 mg of the amino acid lysine to block the herpes virus from reactivation. During outbreaks, increase to as high as 4,000 mg a day, and reduce gradually during the outbreak as the situation looks better. Caution: Do not take lysine for more than six months at a time, because it creates a harmful imbalance with other amino acids. Take more vitamin C to help the healing process. At the onset of an attack, holistic physicians recommend 150 to 1,000 mg an hour to boost the immune system and mute the attack. After blisters emerge, take small amounts of vitamin C throughout the day. Pound the thymus area of the ribcage to increase immune function.

Eating acidophilus yogurt or taking acidophilus capsules with each meal can inhibit cold sores. Dr. Julian Whitaker recommends a product called Herpilyn for prevention and treatment of cold sores. Apply to the lips 2 to 4 times a day during an outbreak. It contains the herb *Melissa officinalis* (lemon balm), which has invaluable antioxidants that strengthen the immune system. An at-home antiviral remedy can be created by placing melissa tea bags directly on the sores. Cold milk compresses also seem to help heal and soothe the lesions.

CONSTIPATION

Water Therapy

To overcome even chronic cases of constipation, adults should drink 2 glasses of cold water first thing in the morning. The cold water provokes peristaltic action in the bowels. Continue to flush and hydrate the system with at least 8 glasses of water during the day. If you are particularly constipated, flush the system by drinking 3 glasses of cold water, one every 10 minutes. Use internal streams of water (an enema) to unblock the system if this doesn't work.

For spastic constipation (cramps), take hot enemas and flood the body with copious amounts of muscle-relaxing chamomile tea.

For chronic constipation it is necessary to tone the abdominal and eliminative organs. With a hand-held shower direct contrast showers of long hot and short cold streams to the abdomen and on occasion to the anus. A long-range, general tone-up for the abdomen is the cold-wet compress covered with a dry towel. Attach the two with a long elastic bandage or cloth. Wear while sleeping, and over the course of a few months it will tone the digestive and eliminative organs. In addition, try an occasional quick dip in a cold bath or a cold lake to stimulate all the organs of elimination.

General Therapy

Check with your physician about possible hydrochloric acid depletion—this mainly occurs in adults over the age of forty or fifty. There are hydrochloride and betaine pills available in health food stores. Do not take them if you have a peptic or stomach ulcer!

Garlic (fresh or in capsules) kills bad bacteria. Acidophilus capsules or cultured yogurt helps establish friendly flora in the intestines. Fibrous food helps move waste material through the bowels, and pectin-rich foods help the bowels to function better. Prunes and figs are excellent natural laxatives. Since constipation can be associated with stress, practice breathing techniques, relaxing mental imagery, and some form of easy exercise such as walking or swimming.

CONTACT LENS PROBLEMS

Water Therapy

Wash hands before inserting contacts, and refrain from touching the inner surface of the lens, which rests against the cornea.

General Therapy

Contact lens wearers frequently complain of dry eyes and irritation. To overcome such problems, wait 20 to 30 minutes after waking up to insert lenses so that the corneas have a chance to return to their normal waking size. Use aerosol deodorants and/or hairsprays well before inserting the lenses. Do not swim with contacts, since contacts, especially soft lenses, absorb chemicals.

COUGHS

Water Therapy

Water in the form of hot steam, compresses, poultices, or liquid is a remarkable way to overcome chest congestion and mucus. Remember to keep the sickroom hydrated with pans of fresh, clean water.

Drink as much water as you can to flush out the system. Hot lemonade (6 washed lemons) laced with 1 tablespoon of honey for each cup is helpful in controlling a cough. Drink this hot lemonade throughout the day. Also sip hot herbal tea with chamomile, thyme, marjoram, and bruised cinnamon, cloves, or aniseed. And of course, there is the age-old elixir:

chicken soup. It not only provides necessary vitamins and protein, but the hot broth breaks up mucus and diminishes the cough.

Salt water is an old standby for colds, cough, and flu. Use it in these two ways: sniffed up each nostril (dissolve a half-teaspoon of salt in a half-glass of water), and as a gargle to soothe a throat made raw from coughing. (Dissolve 1 tablespoon in a glass of water.)

Run a hot shower with the door closed and sit in the bathroom breathing in the steam. Or purchase a steam vaporizer, which emits healing steam for eight hours at a time. Add several drops of tincture of benzoin (from the drugstore) to the well. It leaves a sticky residue, but is wonderfully effective for coughs.

A hot footbath relieves a cough by drawing congestion away from the chest to the feet. This effect is greatly strengthened with the addition of 1 tablespoon powdered mustard seed in the water.

To stimulate the bronchial system, apply a cold wet double compress to the chest. First apply a soft, large wet (wrung out) towel to the chest and cover with a larger, dry towel so that no air penetrates to the wet area. Renew every 30 minutes. This modifies the cough, eases expectoration, relieves labored breathing, and improves chest and general circulation.

Nothing is better for overcoming a resistant cough than the mustard poultice (also called mustard plaster). Set up a large, soft, clean cloth about as large as a man's handkerchief. Combine 1 tablespoon (more for a large person, half for a child) of mustard powder, 4 tablespoons of flour, and 2 tablespoons of tepid water to make a paste. Fold the cloth into an envelope. If the patient has delicate skin, first apply a thin coat of oil or Vaseline. Apply the closed cloth to the chest and back. Keep on sliding the poultice around as the area reddens and blood is released to the surface of the skin. For children, cut the recipe with more flour to make a milder paste.

General Therapy

Zone Therapy as created by the late Dr. William Fitzgerald comes to the rescue of cough victims by pointing out that pressure on the middle of the tongue and/or on the roof of the mouth can deactivate the coughing impulse. Squeezing the uppermost joint of the middle finger is also useful in stopping a fit of coughing. Add hot condiments such as ginger, cayenne pepper, horseradish, or garlic to foods to stimulate expectoration. A series of echinacea treatments (10 days on and 10 days off) will stimulate the immune system.

CRAMPS

Water Therapy

Warm baths relax muscles. During menstrual cramps, run a 6-inch warm-water hip (sitz) bath to increase blood flow to the pelvic region.

Drink plenty of water before, during, and after all athletic activities.

General Therapy

Muscle cramps are most often caused by an imbalance of calcium and magnesium. Ameliorate cramps by supplementing with 1,500 mg of calcium and 750 mg of magnesium. Increase circulation with a vitamin E supplement. Start low with 30 IU and gradually move up to 400 IU. If plagued with cramps, end with 1,000 IU a day. Eat plenty of potassium-rich foods such as bananas, oranges, dark-green vegetables, cornmeal, or kelp. To prevent muscle tightening after a workout, rub pure olive, canola, or flaxseed oil on muscles. Apple cider vinegar splashes on the arms and legs, apple cider vinegar in the bathwater, and apple cider vinegar compresses help to prevent muscle spasms. For menstrual cramps, one week prior to your period, eliminate red meat, caffeine, salt, and junk foods.

DEPRESSION

Water Therapy

Depression is a systemic problem, not a character flaw. One in five women and one in ten men may have some episode of depression during their life. But what causes the changes in biochemistry? Possible causes may include food sensitivity and food allergy; environmental sensitivity from invisible environmental substances, even an infinitesimal gas appliance leak; and a possible internal *Candida* (yeast) infection. Water therapy is an adjunctive approach to depression and can be used to destress, tranquilize, and restore energy.

At times depression takes the form of agitation. Chamomile, St. John's wort tea or tablets, and valerian tablets or tincture help to tranquilize and calm the body. Drops of valerian tincture or a strong chamomile tea may be placed in the bathwater to allay agitation.

We often need to be stimulated out of a depressive mood. Avoid hot baths at this time and concentrate on any of these animating techniques: Before taking a bath, activate the skin by dry brushing, or during the bath vigorously rub the skin with a wet washcloth, sponge, or loofah. Once a week apply a coarse salt friction glow to the shoulders, torso, arms, thighs, and knees. Alternating hot and cold plain or needle-spray showers are also stimulating and restoring to the spirit. Always end alternating showers with a brief cold spray.

Seek out a day spa for a stimulating Swedish massage or a herbal wrap.

General Therapy

Get checked by a clinical ecologist for possible food allergies. Exercise physiologists have determined that vigorous movement for about a half-hour a day produces endorphins, a natural antidepressant and mood lifter. Often something as simple as a spirited walk before breakfast can help dispose of a depression. Other uplifting exercises are swimming and dancing, preferably with a group. Small amounts of Siberian ginseng will increase one's energy and positive mood, and St. John's wort is a prime plant anti-depressant. Watch out for sun exposure when taking St. John's wort—it increases photosensitivity. Various fish contain invaluable omega-3, a substance often deficient in depressed people. Eat salmon, sardines, mackerel, and herring several times a week, or sprinkle ground flaxseed, a substance rich in omega-3, on cereals and salads.

Other procedures that are enormously helpful are hatha yoga breathing techniques and stretching classes; mental imaging that concentrates on positive future incidents; and a variety of meditation techniques. Try to avoid feeling alone and isolated. Join community groups and networks with people who have the same hobbies or share your social, political, or religious interests.

DIABETES

Water Therapy

Diabetes is a disease of the vascular system. Water therapy helps with internal body circulation and should be a daily aid in offsetting damage to the vascular system.

Drinking lots of water decreases the amount of sugar in the system. Drink up to several quarts between meals each day. Hard water with a high mineral content is useful.

Do not apply extreme heat or extreme cold to legs, feet, arms, or hands! However, it is sometimes helpful to apply large hot compresses (always cover this compress with a larger, dry towel) to the upper thighs and groin for short intervals.

Since cold showers increase one's oxidation more than 100 percent, diabetics can try cool showers. The increased oxidation is valuable to diabetics because it prevents some of the secondary skin problems associated with the disease, and also releases the unoxidized sugar through the skin and the kidneys. Naturally the coolness depends on body tolerance, but the water should never be too cold. Occasionally, apply alternate long bursts of warm and short bursts of cool sprays, ending with the cool.

While taking relaxing warm or neutral baths (never too hot!), put a thin layer of oil over the upper extremities and gently massage with about 1 tablespoon of coarse salt dissolved in half a cup of water.

General Therapy

Exercise is vital for diabetics, especially to overcome susceptibility to fatigue. Swedish massage and swimming usually give good results in boosting the circulation. Maintain ideal body weight and control blood sugar by following the appropriate diet under medical supervision. A glucose-insulin tolerance test will help determine whether you should be on a high-complex-carbohydrate diet or a low-carbohydrate (high-protein) diet. Legumes (beans) can be an important part of a high-complex-carbohydrate diet. Keep saturated-fat foods at the lowest level possible. Herring, salmon, mackerel, sardines, oils from vegetables, nuts, and seeds, and capsules of flaxseed, evening primrose, borage, or black currant seed are high in essential omega-3 and omega-6 fatty acids. Some or all of these should be added to the diet. Skin lesions can be effectively treated with vitamin E from a capsule, or aloe vera gel slit from a living plant. To counter diabetic neuropathy, an excruciating nerve pain, purchase one of the several over-the-counter cayenne pepper (capsaicin) ointments. They usually come in two strengths and take about ten days to two weeks to show results. They can also be used for the nerve pain associated with shingles.

Experimental studies show that bruised fenugreek seed tea or debitterized fenugreek seed powder in hot water can often improve glucose tolerance. Two other foods, garlic (or garlic capsules) and onions, act on the cardiovascular system, improve blood lipid levels, and help to lower high blood pressure and high blood sugar levels.

DIARRHEA

ACUTE ATTACK

An unusual flow of wastes (diarrhea) from the body is the natural way the body eliminates toxins in an acute bacterial, viral, or parasitic attack. However, when the diarrhea is so severe that it becomes a menace to recovery, you must stop it. The goal of water therapy is to help the body eliminate the poisons causing the attack.

Stop eating during the attack.

Water Therapy

Since a key problem with diarrhea is the possibility of dehydration, sip water or ice chips constantly. Watch out for evidence of thirst or dry lips or tongue, and drink even more water.

Rice water, made from brown rice, helps to firm up loose stools and replace the body's B vitamins, which are eliminated with the diarrhea. Make rice water by combining half a cup of brown rice to 3 cups of boiling water. Simmer for 45 minutes. Strain out the rice, which can be eaten later, and drink the remaining rice water.

To Avoid Dehydration: Avoid the effects of severe dehydration with this recipe: Dissolve 1 tablespoon of salt, 4 tablespoons of sugar, and a half-cup of apple cider vinegar in 2 quarts or 1 liter of water. Sip throughout the day.

It strongly helps to cleanse the lower colon with a warm enema. Many people find this puzzling. Why use an enema to evacuate material when there is so much material emerging on its own? Repeated hot rectal irrigations cause the kidney to function even when drugs fail. And an enema will bring instant relief because it rids the body of toxic diarrhea-inducing substances. This enema may be repeated frequently during the day if necessary.

If a child has a severe attack of diarrhea, flush the anal area with cold sterile water after each bowel movement. If food poisoning is suspected, try a strong, non-decaffeinated coffee enema, but only for healthy adults, because this is a very potent enema.

Ease the pain of the diarrhea by applying a large hot, moist compress to the stomach area twice a day, or alternate hot and cool compresses to the area. Apple cider vinegar may be added to each compress to accelerate the healing process.

Facilitate a quick recovery by boosting circulation in the body through dry brushing or a rough wet washcloth friction rub.

Drink ginger tea to counter any nausea associated with the diarrhea.

To Stop Diarrhea: If it is an emergency, a normally healthy person can take a sitz (sit) bath in 6 to 8 inches of cold water for a few seconds, gradually increasing the time up to 10 minutes in temperatures of 40°F to 50°F. A half-cup of apple cider vinegar can be added to the sitz bath. During the sitz bath, place towels on the chest and back to protect from drafts. As part of the treatment, massage the upper body through the towels. After the bath, again rub the entire body with a rough towel. This sitz bath is not for infants, sickly children, feeble or elderly patients, pregnant women, or those with heart problems.

Cooked carrot soup (which is high in pectin), cooked barley soup, or rice soup are enormously helpful in reducing watery stools, and are easily tolerated by children and adults alike.

To Control Pain and Reduce Vomiting: You can inhibit pain and vomiting somewhat by placing a hot apple cider vinegar and water compress on the abdomen.

Children (Chronic Attacks): When children have chronic attacks of diarrhea, detective work is imperative. Check for possible food triggers, food sensitivities, or a chronic stress situation that should be remedied. If the child is normally healthy, try the following two water therapy techniques for strengthening the child's digestive and immune system. Do not do this with infants.

In a draft-free bathroom, quickly place the child in a cold half bath for a few seconds at a time. Dry him or her immediately with a large towel. Do this every day for the first week after an attack. Then use these baths every other day.

For one to several weeks after an attack, to help tone the internal organs, apply the cold abdominal compress technique using either cold or warm water or warm diluted apple cider vinegar in the compress. Apply a fresh compress each time.

General Therapy

At the first indication of diarrhea, take 1 to 2 tablets of activated charcoal. Charcoal absorbs toxic and poisonous material in the gut. Repopulate the invaded gut with capsules, liquid, or powdered *Lactobacillus acidophilus,* and *Lactobacillus bulgaricus,* both of which combat diarrhea-inducing bacteria *E. coli,* salmonella, streptococci, and shigella. These capsules can be obtained in a health food store. Is yogurt good enough? Only some brands of yogurt contain live cultures. Take garlic capsules for their antibiotic impact, especially against gram-negative bacteria. The pectin in an apple is quite useful. Peel and scrape the apple to release the pectin. Also eat small pieces of banana or blueberries. The following food products can be used as teas and can be very beneficial: dried blueberries or blueberry extract, extract of peppermint or peppermint, chamomile or raspberry leaf. A few grains of cayenne pepper in water or tea often stops queasiness. When the diarrhea is cleared up, replace the flushed-out enzymes with fresh papaya or papaya juice, fresh pineapple or pineapple juice, or mild, diluted lemon juice.

DIGESTIVE PROBLEMS

DIGESTIVE AID

Carminative waters, an old-fashioned European digestive aid that is inexpensive and easy to prepare, is wonderful. Add 1 teaspoon each of chamomile, fennel, caraway, coriander, and bitter orange peel to 1 cup of hot water. Let the mixture stand, and drink hot or cold.

STOMACH CRAMPS

Stomach pain that is a result of overeating can be relieved by standing for 10 to 15 minutes under a relatively hot shower until the stomach area turns red. You can also achieve similar relief by applying hot moist compresses to the area, followed by a poultice of chopped raw onion or pulped cabbage. These poultices reduce internal fermentation and subdue the cramps.

STOMACH SPASMS

An effective remedy for acute spasms is this two-part cold and hot application. First, slightly oil the abdomen and the area of the back between the shoulders. Place a small, wet, cold, wrung-out towel on these two areas. Place a piping-hot compress or a hot water bottle over the abdomen and shoulder area. Keep the application on for about a half-hour.

INDIGESTION

Whenever you have the discomfort of indigestion, it is useful to take frequent neutral-temperature baths (well below body temperature) for 30 minutes at a time. If possible, add pine essence or strong melissa tea to the bathwater. Such neutral baths relieve the tension caused by the indigestion and also activate internal digestive secretions.

There are two long-range water therapies for chronic indigestion: (1) Tread in 6 inches of cold water while holding on to the bath bar. (2) Take a brief few seconds cold dip in the bath once a day and follow this heroic gesture with a hot compress or hot water bottle to both the abdomen and the shoulders. End with cold compresses to the two areas.

Dr. Ronald L. Hoffman, in his book *7 Weeks to a Settled Stomach,* suggests taking some hot, tonic, or aromatic bitter herbs to soothe a stomachache. For indigestion, Hoffman suggests eating small slices of raw ginger. A shortcut that works in our house is to buy sweetened crystallized ginger and wash off all the sugar. This makes a quick, healthy dessert, too. Chamomile, peppermint, and raspberry leaf tea are also good for indigestion and stomach cramps. All digestive tonics are made up of a variety of herbs such as gentian, catnip, fennel, lavender, star anise, cayenne, cardamom, angelica, and prickly ash berries. Use any of these as a strong tea.

Whenever I'm in Switzerland, France, or Germany I make sure to pick up a bottle of Melisana, a concentration of the bitter herb melissa. It is an ancient Carmelite remedy created by nuns and a wonderful palliative for an upset stomach. Look for the bottle with the emblem of three Carmelite nuns.

DUODENAL ULCERS

Several long-term stratagems will eventually help relieve the pain of duodenal ulcers. Every day dry-brush the body, then take a long, relaxing bath. During each bath, friction rub the shoulders, torso, arms, legs, and thighs with a rough washcloth. Several times a week, alternate these baths with brief hot and even briefer cold sitz baths. As often as possible at other times of the day, use directed cold shower sprays to various parts of the body.

DRY MOUTH

Saliva is essential to the health of the mouth, especially since bacteria increase when saliva is in short supply. Further, an extremely dry mouth causes problems both in eating and in swallowing. A dry mouth can be an indication of other health problems, so check it out with your physician.

Water Therapy

There are a variety of saliva replacement sprays available in pharmacies. Experiment until you find one that helps you best.

Carry bottled water with you at all times to refresh the mouth and temporarily replace missing saliva. When eating, have cool water on hand to add to hot drinks like soup, coffee, or tea.

Cayenne pepper stimulates the saliva. Add tiny amounts to food or tea. Other special stimulants that can be added to foods and drinks are drops of echinacea tincture, green tea, ginger ale, and ginger tea.

Prepare a home herbal mouthwash with one glass of water, 1 tablespoon of vodka, 5 drops of tincture of myrrh, and 5 drops of tincture of goldenseal. Use on occasion to cleanse and decontaminate the mouth.

General Therapy

It is essential to visit a dentist on a regular basis, because without essential saliva, teeth tend to deteriorate quickly. Include both vitamin C and beta carotene supplements in your daily diet. Eat several citrus fruits each day, as well as yellow and orange vegetables.

EAR PROBLEMS

EAR INFECTION

Water Therapy

Hot moist compresses help to relieve the pain of an inflammation of the outer ear. Alternate hot and cold compresses increase the absorption of inflammatory deposits.

Hot salt bag applications will relieve acute ear pain. Place 2 pounds coarse salt in a cotton pillowcase or soft old towel and heat the salt bag in the oven until it is very hot. Wrap in an old soft cloth or pillowcase to prevent burning, and lie down with the afflicted ear against the salt bag. If there is pus or catarrhal blockage in the ear, the salt will draw the waste material out and relieve the pressure-induced pain.

What we often need with an ear infection is to divert inflammation from the ear area. Fortunately, water therapy has several ways to divert heat and inflammation from one area to another. Choices are foot wrappings, foot compresses, hot footbaths, which will divert blood flow to the feet, or a comfortable cold double throat compress, which brings heat to the area of the throat. Dip a folded dishcloth into cold water or apple cider vinegar, wring it out, and pin it around the throat. Immediately place a wool scarf or fabric piece over the cold wet compress and pin it. The body will immediately send heat to the area of the throat, and ease the earache at the same time.

At the first twinge of a problem, swab the ear with a cotton stick dipped into equal parts of apple cider vinegar and rubbing alcohol. This combination is also excellent for preventing the itchiness and flakiness of swimmer's ear.

James Duke in *Green Pharmacy* suggests combining 1 capsule garlic oil with 4 parts vegetable oil to treat a bacterial or fungal ear infection. (Never use herbal ear drops if you have reason to believe the eardrum is perforated.) Mullein is another reliable, ancient healing ear oil. Heat and apply on a wad of absorbent cotton placed in the outer ear. This can be used for both adults and children.

General Therapy

Ear infections are a common and painful part of childhood. The usual medical practice is to treat middle ear infections with antibiotics. Although this is quite necessary in crisis situations, it doesn't address the cause of repeated ear infections. According to the distinguished nutritionist-physician Dr. Alan Gaby, the most important preventive action against recurrent ear infections in children is an investigation of possible food allergies. According to Gaby, food allergies can cause congestion in the eustachian tubes of the inner ear. There the fluid buildup is a breeding ground for bacteria. The most common food allergies are to dairy products, sugar, corn (corn syrup is hidden in most prepared foods), eggs, citrus fruits, and chocolate. Particularly watch out for the effect of sugar on the immune system because it weakens a child's ability to fight infections. The first thing to eliminate is any cow's milk–based food. Once the infection clears up, you may reintroduce one food at a time to see which one the child tolerates well. Dr. Leo Galland, a holistic physician formerly with the Gesell Institute, recommends giving the child 1 to 2 teaspoons of flaxseed oil daily. Some children adore the taste of this oil. If they resist taking it internally, or if the child is very young, rub this flaxseed oil directly on the scalp and skin, usually about one hour before the bath. Store the oil in the refrigerator to prevent rancidity. Galland also suggests supplementing the child's diet with 500 mg or up to 1,000 mg of vitamin C. In any case, the point of tolerance for vitamin C, whether taken by an adult or by a child, is when diarrhea occurs. At that point the body is taking in enough vitamin C.

EAR WAX

Dissolve ear wax by applying a few drops of warm, not hot, vegetable or mullein oil in the ear. Afterwards gently flush the ear with warm water in a bulb syringe. Keep the head upright. Drain out the water and wax by turning the head sideways and down. Instead of the oil, hydrogen peroxide 5% can be gently swabbed or dripped into the ear, then flushed out with warm water.

MENIERE'S DISEASE

Water Therapy

People with Meniere's disease appear to have severe vertigo. Since fluid accumulation is damaging with this problem, as is increased volume and pressure in the inner ear, utilize natural herbal and food diuretics to curb water retention. Choose one or several of these: parsley tea, asparagus or asparagus tincture, watermelon, corn silk tea, or small doses of vitamin B$_6$. To further reduce fluid retention, lessen salt intake. Also see "Edema" in "Heart Problems" section.

General Therapy

Avoid nicotine or any other substance that might trigger nausea. Check with an ear, nose, and throat specialist for possible polyps in the nose, as they can cause this problem.

ECZEMA

Water Therapy

Frequent neutral-temperature half-baths, cold sponges to the body, and alternate hot and cold showers directed to the thighs and upper chest are excellent therapies for toning the body.

Relieve the itching of an eczema attack with a bath containing colloidal oatmeal (Aveeno).

Apply chamomile tea bags to lesions to soothe the eczema.

General Therapy

Aloe vera gel from a houseplant (test it first before slathering it on) is a great instant ointment to offset the itching. Stinging nettle or chickweed ointment are also beneficial. Calendula homeopathic ointment is very healing for the scales and itching. Burdock tablets are used in two ways. Take internally to help detoxify the body, and apply some powder to the lesions for scaly eczema.

Vegetable juices produce intense infusions of needed vitamins, and also flush the system. The following juices are helpful for eczema: beet, carrot, celery, cucumber, endive, spinach, and parsley. Many persons who suffer from eczema need an additional intake of vegetable oils and/or vitamin F.

The nutritional expert Dr. Alan Gaby feels that appropriate nutritional therapy eliminates the need for potentially dangerous steroid therapy in the treatment of eczema. Many eczema patients appear to lack the ability to utilize essential fatty acids (EFAs), but these can be supplemented by oils such as sunflower, safflower, flaxseed, black currant seed, borage, or evening primrose. Many are available in capsule form and should be taken every day, usually for the entire lifetime of an eczema patient. It is important to remember that long-term use of EFA supplements increases one's need for vitamin E. Supplements that will alleviate adult flareups are kelp tablets, B-complex tablets, vitamin E, and zinc. Zinc is essential for the production of the digestive acid hydrochloric acid, and for its known ability to convert essential fatty acids into anti-inflammatory substances. Add only a minimal dose of zinc to the diet.

Foods can trigger eczema attacks. Try eliminating dairy products, eggs, tomatoes, and citrus fruits, then reintroduce each food one at a time. Watch out for a reaction, and remove any offending food from the diet.

Cell salt therapy is most useful. Start with ferrum phos. 6x at the onset of any attack.

Eczema is such a variable problem that you must experiment with the general treatments to find which ones work the best for you. Oatmeal soaps and colloidal oatmeal washes are often helpful. Applications of vitamin E oil can help overcome the dryness. Napier's (Edinburgh) Slippery Elm soap helps some people and Nelson's (London) Calendula and Hamamelis Hand and Skin Lotion has also been used successfully.

Eczema patients may occasionally use valerian to calm the nerves. The Bach Flower Remedies, which help change your emotional state, are also effective.

ELIMINATION

Water Therapy

Water helps elimination in three distinct ways.

Drink 1 to 2 quarts of water and/or diuretic herbal teas to promote fluid elimination through the kidneys and bladder. Watermelon flesh or juice, asparagus in vegetable form or tincture, tea of corn silk, and parsley soup or tea will stimulate the flow of urine.

A long, hot bath will induce perspiration to form and exude through the pores of the skin. In particular, hayflower extract, oatstraw, or fennel tea will strongly detoxify the system. This type of elimination can also be encouraged by skin brushing. Such skin stroking can easily be accomplished with a special soft brush for dry-brushing the skin, loofah rubs, energetic wet washcloth massages, or kneading coarse salt plus water on the torso and limbs.

Internal irrigation with a warm enema, or a professional colonic, will extract hardened waste material from the colon. For about half a century, some nonallopathic healers have also advised detoxifying the body with strong coffee enemas. This has been used in some alternative cancer treatments.

Fresh vegetable juices are generally effective in refreshing the cells and in toning and cleansing the body. Organic beet powder added to pure water is especially purifying.

FATIGUE

Water Therapy

For Instant Revival: Hold the wrists and/or ankles under cold running water.

Restore energy, slake thirst, and avoid dehydration with a series of slowly sipped cups of pure water. Drinking water throughout the day will replenish flagging energy.

Other Quick Water Energizers: Prior to taking a shower or bath, generously splash apple cider vinegar over the shoulders, torso, arms, and legs. This restores the acid pH covering of the skin and helps to replenish waning energy.

Snatch a quick alternate hot-cold, hot-cold percussion shower using long bursts of hot, short torrents of cold, ending with a cold splash. This will restore energy immediately. Another instant booster is a series of alternate long hot and short cold foot splashes. Afterwards, rub each area of the sole, sides, and top of the foot. Since one section of the foot is believed to control the kidney area, this helps facilitate the return of energy.

Take a 3-second dunk in hot water (a brief immersion in hot is very stimulating), or a long, leisurely warm-to-hot bath. At the end of the bath dribble in cold water to offset the depleting action of the heat. Complete the restoration of energy with a salt-glow friction rub.

Hot drinks with herbs will also lift the spirits. Add a pinch of Siberian ginseng powder, ginger extract, or cayenne powder to these teas: peppermint, melissa, or fennel. It will greatly help to consume an extra vitamin C and calcium citrate tablet as well as a chlorophyll tablet.

Ever wonder why washing one's hair restores energy flow and makes one feel better? The scalp, neck, and face contain dozens of key body trigger points. Stimulating this area restarts blocked energy points. During the shampoo, as if holding a ball, drum your taut fingers over the scalp, neck, and shoulders and energetically tap all areas of the face. Also thoroughly rub the lobes of each ear. In the Chinese system of acupuncture, the ear is a microcosm of the body, so pulling, rubbing, and stroking each speck of outer ear tissue also restores blocked energy.

Tired, dry eyes signal a tired body. Restore normally tired eyes with compresses over closed eyes. Use either plain water, witch hazel extract, eyebright tea or slices of cucumber. For dry eyes, apply Refresh, nonpreservative, over-the-counter eyedrops that come in individual one-use containers.

General Therapy

Shallow breathing denotes a sustained lack of oxygen to the lungs. Practice taking deep breaths twice every hour. A never-fail restoration of energy can be accomplished by lying down with the head much lower than the feet; try this on a slantboard, which you can find in catalogs. This reversal of gravity is amazingly effective. While lying this way, cover your closed eyes with cooling slices of cucumber or soothing cotton pads soaked in witch hazel. Another energizing activity is the "thymus thump," which activates the gland and brings energy to the whole body: Simply pound on your thymus gland, located in the center of your ribcage. Do it 3 to 4 times a day to reduce the effects of stress.

For persistent fatigue check possible food sensitivities, especially to wheat, corn, milk, and eggs, although any food eaten regularly may be an offender. One possible indication of such sensitivity is puffiness of the eyelids and fullness and discoloration of the eyes. Work with a medical nutritionist to uncover possible nutritional deficiencies.

FEVER

Water Therapy

Water therapy is nature's remarkable answer to reducing the symptoms of fever.

Here are the outstanding examples of what water can do:

Drinking: The more cool water one drinks, the more a fever can be decreased.

Irrigation: A tap-water enema instantly cools the lower part of the body.

Cold Baths: They quickly reduce even dangerous fevers.

Hot Drinks, Hot Baths, Compresses: These plus encasing oneself in blankets stimulate the largest organ, the skin, to secrete perspiration.

Diuretic Foods and Drinks: They have the power to activate the kidneys and bladder to eliminate excess fluid as urine.

Even when the cause of the fever is unknown, water therapies should be used immediately, especially in conjunction with vitamin C therapy and when needed, antibacterial drugs. One interesting illustration of the power of water therapy to reduce an excessively high fever occurred during a 1976 bicentennial celebration when a then-unknown epidemic killed many Pennsylvania Legionnaires who had just returned from their convention in Philadelphia. The ex-soldiers suffered raging 108° fevers and pneumonia-like symptoms. Most died, except the one who was lucky enough to have been treated with both "old-fashioned" water therapy and an antibiotic.

The foremost antifever strategy is to drink liquids. Fever can be reduced from one-half to 2 degrees by drinking 2 to 3 pints of cold water within a 10-minute period, although this time can be extended.

High, extreme, and dangerous fevers require more water than ordinary fevers. Patients must drink between 6 to 7 quarts of liquid in 24 hours to have an effect on near-fatal fevers. These drinks will reduce the fever and quench the thirst of the patient: sage tea, apple cider vinegar and water, raspberry vinegar and water (in a pinch combine raspberry jam, apple cider vinegar, and water), lemon juice and water, and peppermint tea.

A cool tap-water enema will cool the body internally and also help the healing process when it evacuates waste materials. If further evacuation is necessary, utilize a gentle herbal laxative such as Inner Clean. Acidophilus powder or capsules are useful to restore beneficial bacteria to the gut.

Cold baths at this time work well! They have even worked during cholera epidemics. Even if it seems heroic—do it. It need only be a brief dip into the cold water to help. Sometimes it helps a small infant or toddler if a loving, relaxed adult gets into the bath at the same time. Immediately towel-rub the patient dry. If the patient is too feeble, too young, or too large to move, some of the same effect is accomplished using vigorous wet washcloth friction rubs. To further reduce the fever, apple cider vinegar or raspberry vinegar may be added to the water. Cover the patient completely and only rub one uncovered area at a time.

Baths in pine extract help to reduce fever.

Induce perspiration with hot drinks such as sage tea and by wrapping the patient in a wool blanket. At the same time use a cool, wet compress on the head. Should the patient complain of the heat from being encased in the blanket, soak a pair of cotton socks in apple cider vinegar, wring them out, and place on the feet. This indirect therapy not only reduces the body heat, but also draws congestion away from the head area. Hot compresses to the chest and buttocks will also induce body perspiration, as will a steaming hot bath, especially if it contains Epsom salts or hayflower extract. Do not use Epsom salts for a child, the frail elderly, or those with a chronic disease or heart trouble. Once the perspiration is induced, keep on daubing the forehead and the body to remove perspiration. Sponge the perspiration off with cool water or apple cider vinegar. The patient should be tired and ready for a good sleep.

Use drinks containing natural diuretics to stimulate the kidneys to eliminate excess fluids. Teas of parsley, asparagus, or chunks of watermelon are easily obtained foods that are natural diuretics. Horsetail and corn silk as well as other herbs are excellent diuretics.

For a dangerous fever, relax the head, heart, and respiratory system with a series of hot sage tea footbaths. During each bath apply continuous damp, cold compresses to the back of the neck. Wrap the patient in a wet, cold cotton sheet.

FLABBY MUSCLES

Water Therapy

A wonderful and easy way to tone up flabby muscles and listless nerves is to stimulate the body with a sheet bath. This sheet bath requires a warm sheet (warm it over a radiator or on an electric pad) and another sheet soaked in cold water and wrung out so that it is not dripping. You will need someone to help you with the massage.

Stand naked while your helper wraps the wet sheet tightly around you. She or he then rubs your body through the sheet with long and vigorous strokes down the length of the arms, body, and legs. When the helper feels surface warmth from your body through the sheet, she or he discards the wet sheet and wraps the preheated sheet around you in the same way, continuing to rub with the same strokes until you are completely dried.

The sheet bath only takes about 4 to 6 minutes, and quickly brings a sensation of liveliness to the body. A series of these sheet baths once a week will help to restore body tone to those who are convalescing from an illness.

FLU

Influenza viruses are potent, airborne, highly contagious, and do not respond to antibiotic therapy. What to do when a virus hits? Drink copious amounts of water to cleanse the system of toxins, and use every known perspiration-inducing technique to force additional toxins out through the skin. Water healing techniques can strengthen resistance and thus boost immunity, shorten the infectious period, and offer needed support during convalescence after a flu attack.

During the flu season wash your hands often! While the virus is airborne, it is most often transmitted via the hands near the nose. So keep your hands away from your nose and face.

To prevent dehydration and boost elimination through perspiration, drink liberal amounts of water.

Prevent infection by viruses and bacteria by sluicing a salt solution up each nostril—first thing in the morning and several times a day.

Cinnamon, especially in oil form, is an ancient remedy to prevent flu. It can be used at the onset of any epidemic. A potent antiflu remedy is 5 drops of cinnamon oil in 1 tablespoon of water, consumed several times a day before a flu attack. Less powerful but still effective is a bruised cinnamon stick (bruising releases the volatile oil) added to a half-cup of boiling water. Steep and drink.

Water Therapy

When the flu strikes, reduce any fever by drinking glass after glass of pure water. Each ounce you drink will reduce the fever. See the "Fever" section.

Cayenne pepper is a famous flu chaser. Add a pinch to any herbal tea. A terrific antiflu remedy beloved by many (and abhorred by some—it is strong stuff!) is a combination of salt, cayenne, apple cider vinegar, and boiled water, or if a stomach buffer is needed, hot chamomile tea instead of the boiled water. Combine 1 tablespoon each of coarse or sea salt and cayenne pepper powder, add to 1 cup of boiling water (or chamomile tea). Cool the preparation. Add a quarter- to a half-cup of apple cider vinegar (depending on the sturdiness of one's digestive system). Place in a labeled bottle. Store in the refrigerator. Drink in quarter-teaspoon doses every few hours before and during the flu epidemic. A word of warning: Some of my students thought this was the best thing that ever happened to them. Others hated it.

Ginseng powder added to a herbal tea will hasten healing and add immune system support.

Think of hot liquids as an invaluable asset in fighting the flu. The following as well as the cayenne pepper and ginseng are powerful aids: immune-boosting echinacea tea; elderflower as a tea, or combined with peppermint and yarrow to induce and promote needed perspiration; hot lemonade with honey; or great-grandma's standby—hot chicken soup, because even its vapors help to clear nasal passages.

Other herbal teas useful for the flu are slippery elm bark for cough, fever, and sore throat; eucalyptus for congestion and cough; horehound and cherry bark for cough. Sage tea will increase kidney function and help to expel quantities of extra fluid from the body.

During the flu it is imperative to perspire freely, but not become chilled. Take hot detoxification baths, which should also induce sleep: half or full hot baths to relieve body aches and induce perspiration. At the same time as the bath, apply a cold compress to the head and drink either hot lemonade, hot pineapple juice, or any of the above herbal tea drinks. To increase the impact of these hot baths, add 1 cup of apple cider vinegar, 1 cup of Epsom salts, or a half-cup of pine extract to the bathwater. At various times during the day after sleeping and before or after taking a hot bath, stimulate the heart by applying a series of cold compresses to the heart area.

Optional: The following morning after the first detoxification bath, relieve some of the aching of the back and limbs with simultaneous hot applications to the legs and to the back and spine. Conclude this treatment with a cold friction massage.

During convalescence follow all these treatments with tonic water therapy measures such as a cold friction massage to increase circulation and healing from within, a cold towel rub, or a series of alternate hot and then cold spray showers to the spine and the legs. Always end with the cold application.

Whenever possible, further detoxify the body with an enema to cleanse the internal digestive and eliminative system.

This is "advanced" water healing: Make sure there are no drafts in the room. Prepare a twin-size cotton sheet; fresh garlic thoroughly mashed into a small amount of Vaseline; additional Vaseline; and a large woolen blanket. Wet and wring out the cotton sheet. Wind it around the patient, but before turning the ends of the sheet up around the feet, quickly coat the feet with Vaseline (it has just the right viscosity) and "paint" the soles of the feet (no other part!) with the mashed garlic in Vaseline. Cover the feet and the rest of the body with the sheet and cover the wet sheet with a larger wool blanket. This sheet arrangement helps the body to perspire and shed the virus. The garlic foot "paint" can often turn the tide in this or any other serious disease.

While the body temperature is elevated, the patient should drink fresh juices and forgo solid foods, particularly proteins and fats. Liquid intake should be greater than normal. The best juices are orange, grapefruit, diluted bilberry or blueberry, black currant, and grape. Occasionally alternate with some beet juice to clear the system. If the liver appears to be affected, drink carrot juice instead of fruit juices.

Whenever possible sponge and friction-rub the body with apple cider vinegar or raspberry vinegar washes. This will help bring down the fever. However, if the fever is raging, conduct this instant temperature-reducing strategy: Plunge the patient for a few seconds into a full bath of warm to cool water. Towel dry immediately! Make sure there are no drafts in the room. Such an immersion will also help the patient fall into a restorative sleep. (Do not use for an infant or a feeble invalid.)

If the patient still maintains a fever, apply a cold compress to the calves to make the feverish patient more comfortable and to promote easier sleep.

Maintain oral hygiene—brush teeth and gums. Use the toothbrush to remove any coating from the tongue.

Reduce waste materials in the body with a brief warm enema and a herbal laxative. An activated charcoal tablet is useful at this time to further absorb and discard internal toxins.

General Therapy

Homeopathic medicines are very effective against the flu. There are many such remedies. Oscillococcinum, an impossible to pronounce homeopathic remedy, available in every health food store, is exceptionally helpful if taken at the onset of exposure. It can arrest a flu attack before it starts. Keep some in the medicine chest, glove compartment, briefcase, pocketbook, and office desk! During the flu season definitely increase the intake of vitamin C. Sleep in a well-ventilated room under warm covers. Practice deep breathing to cleanse lungs and tonify the pulmonary system. Air the sickroom frequently. The patient should be well covered and the room should be maintained at a pleasantly cool temperature.

FOOD POISONING

The best way of dealing with food poisoning is by avoiding it. This requires vigilance in the preparation and storage of foods. Use hot soapy water to wash used cutting board and knives, and wash the area clean after any food preparation.

Water Therapy

At the slightest hint of a problem, take a tap-water enema or a prepared enema from the drugstore to cleanse the lower bowel of potentially dangerous substances. Drink some water and swallow an activated charcoal tablet to absorb and eject food poisons, and further eliminate recently eaten food and the potential poison with a mild herbal laxative tablet such as Inner Clean or Swiss Kriss. If you need to vomit the food up, drink some warm salted water or place two fingers toward the back of the throat.

Melisana, the ancient Carmelite nuns' remedy imported from Germany, quickly restores the body. Herbal teas help to relieve food poisoning. Try peppermint tea with a pinch of cayenne pepper. The peppermint is a carminative, and the cayenne pepper is an alterative, which should stimulate and rebalance the system. Chamomile tea will soothe the stomach, relieve nausea, and act as an antiseptic. Add bruised cloves, bruised cinnamon sticks, or shaved ginger to these and other herbal drinks. Ginger is the herb for overcoming nausea and stomach distress. Make a tea with ginger slices, or wash off the sugar on crystallized ginger and add to herbal teas.

FOOT PROBLEMS

ACHING FEET AND LEGS

Water Therapy

Those whose jobs require long hours of standing find that their feet are often swollen and fatigued. Try this extraordinary water therapy wrap for a few evenings before bed, and soon the foot tiredness will disappear. First soak white potato slices in 1 quart of cold water. In a double boiler heat 2 cups of salt. Wash and soak the feet in the potato water. Immediately afterwards, wrap the feet in a cloth containing the hot salt. Repeat for several days in a row.

BLISTER

Water Therapy

At the very first indication of a blister, rub with an ice cube.

General Therapy

Avoid letting the feet get wet and sweaty. Wear cotton socks or footies under other socks to prevent friction. Keep Band-Aids handy for your foot's hot spots.

BUNIONS

Water Therapy

Experiment with both hot and cold therapy, because the reaction varies from person to person.

Whirlpool therapy increases circulation. Soak the feet in hot Epsom salt footbaths.

Reduce swelling of the feet with witch hazel soaks or compresses, or relieve pain by dissolving 4 tablets of homeopathic arnica 6x under the tongue, and externally applying arnica ointment or compresses of arnica dissolved in water.

General Therapy

Exercise the toes by picking up marbles or by rolling your foot over a small round bottle again and again. Try this exercise to stretch and subdue stiffness and inflexibility of the foot: Sit in a chair. Lift one foot at a time and make circles with the toes to the right and to the left. Repeat with the other foot.

To restore a toe to a normal position, tape along the toe with a 1-inch strip of adhesive, and gently stretch and pull the toe into a normal and straightened position. A special nighttime bunion splint recommended by podiatrists is available in both men or women's shoe sizes. Try Comfort Corner, at 1-800-442-8730.

Many patients have success with acupuncture treatments to overcome the pain.

BURNING FEET

Water Therapy

Create your own foot coolers with cold witch hazel, peppermint, or lemon juice dips. Also massage with any of these refreshing and healing oils: lemon, pine, peppermint, lavender, eucalyptus, or wintergreen.

COLD FEET

Water Therapy

For long-range help in promoting better circulation, utilize these showers and/or footbaths.

1. Alternate (contrast) 3-minute hot and 1½-minute cold showers to the body, but especially to the soles of the feet. Always end with a cold splash! Repeat each sequence several times. Dry with a rough towel.

2. Prepare strong hot and cold thyme tea or pine or juniper extract and add to a 2- to 3-minute hot and cold footbath.
3. Use lukewarm water to warm up cold hands and feet. Place cold hands under the armpits to warm them up.

General Therapy

Protect yourself from exposure to cold. Wear warm socks and gloves as well as waterproof boots. Those with cold feet usually respond to gradual increased vitamin E therapy. Start with a low dose of 30 IU and move upward. Ask your doctor about using the herb *Ginkgo biloba*.

Allergy Elimination: For 4 to 6 weeks eliminate caffeine, chocolate, peanuts and peanut butter, and aged cheese from your diet. If as a result of this elimination your hands or feet feel less cold, one of the foods may be the cause of the problem. To find out which one, replace them one at a time.

CORNS

Water Therapy

Soak the feet in warm water for 15 minutes each day. Rub the softened tissue with a mild pumice stone.

FOOT ODOR

Water Therapy

Wash and sponge your feet with apple cider vinegar each morning. Dry thoroughly. Whenever possible during the day, wash feet to discourage the formation of bacteria. Sponge off with rubbing alcohol.

As often as possible soak the feet in apple cider vinegar and water and/or horsetail herb tea, which is high in silica. Conclude each soaking with an alcohol sponging or a lemon juice rinse.

General Therapy

People with strong foot odor often need additional intake of B vitamins. Take a potent daily multivitamin as well as an additional 50 milligrams of a

B-complex vitamin in the morning and evening. For habitually smelly, per-spiring feet, or any other offensive sweat, take three silica 6x homeopathic tablets twice a day. Purchase dozens of white cotton socks and have several changes of shoes. Create air spaces in your shoes by wearing two pairs of cotton socks. Change socks and shoes in the middle of the day. Rinse the socks in boric acid and water and let them air dry.

FLAT FEET

Water Therapy

Use alternate long bursts of hot and short bursts of cold sprays to relieve foot pain.

Soak feet in hot mustard powder or an Epsom salt footbath. End with a short blast of cold water. Wipe feet.

General Therapy

This problem may be congenital. It generally shows by age 8 to 15. A later onset may result from standing on concrete, standing too long at work, or running.

HAMMERTOES

Water Therapy

A 15-minute warm-water soak will soften hardened tissue and corns that form on a hammertoe.

General Therapy

If this problem starts in adulthood, it may be caused by improperly fitted shoes. It is also associated with corns, calluses, excess weight, tight short tendons, arthritis, and diabetes. If it is a result of poor posture, seek out an Alexander or Feldenkreis teacher to relearn how to stand, walk, and sit. Sometimes the pain of hammertoes can be alleviated with constant deep massage to the feet and the shortened tendon. The feet tend to get larger with age and spread wider as the day goes on. Therefore, always buy shoes late in the day. Walk barefoot as often as possible, especially on the grass and outdoors on uneven land. Get rid of tight, narrow, pointed-toe shoes. Purchase special toe cushions to relieve friction and pressure on the toe tips. One source: Comfort Corner, 1-800-735-4994 for right or left foot cushions or single or double toe straighteners.

PERSPIRATION (EXCESSIVE)

Water Therapy

Soak the feet each day for a few minutes in a strong hayflower extract or fennel tea footbath.

To help control excessive perspiration, drink diuretic teas to purify the kidneys: corn silk, buchu, parsley, uva ursi herb teas, or watermelon or asparagus.

SWOLLEN FEET

Water Therapy

Use the same treatment as for aching feet. For swollen feet, one can also combine either fennel or hayflower tea and coarse salt in a footbath. Such footbaths also relieve hot, burning feet. European village healers often advised wrapping swollen feet in cloths dipped in cold hayflower extract or tea once a day for 15 minutes.

FROSTBITE

Frostbite is the destruction of the skin by freezing.

Water Therapy

Rush the victim to the hospital. If this is not possible, rewarm a frostbitten limb in high-temperature water. The U.S. Navy says water at 102°F to 105°F will bring excellent results. Because there may be tissue damage if the thawing is too slow or too fast, use a thermometer to monitor the process. If you don't have a thermometer, see page 70.

Another technique is to keep the frostbitten limb covered with a wool or flannel blanket and warm all other parts of the body. Create maximum circulation by rubbing the limb vigorously. In 30 minutes, a flush usually returns to the skin. The thawed tissues can then be soaked in a whirlpool bath for 20 minutes once or twice a day until the healing is complete.

For children, wrap a compress that has been soaked in neutral water and strained hayflower tea over the affected part. Cover the wet compress with a dry cloth.

Take a series of hand or footbaths with one-quarter vinegar and three-quarters cold water.

General Therapy

During very cold weather, always wear a hat. An uncovered head quickly gives away body heat. Wear mittens instead of gloves. Wear long johns, wool sweaters, and other warm clothing. Wet clothing, fatigue, and a couple of drinks too many can make you more susceptible to frostbite.

GALLBLADDER SYMPTOMS

Water Therapy

In the past, bitter herb teas such as wormwood were successfully used to relieve gallbladder symptoms. However, the tea must be taken sparingly, and for no longer than 3 to 4 weeks. One shortcut is to use either Cinzano or Martini, Italian "digestive" aperitifs that contain just enough of the bitter herbs to aid gallbladder and dyspepsia symptoms. Sip slowly in 1-ounce (shot glass size) portions.

GOUT

Gout is a type of arthritis caused by crystallized uric acid (urate) buildup in the joints, a problem that occurs when urate, a metabolic waste, is not properly expelled and becomes concentrated in the urine. These elevated levels of urate are caused by an excessively rich diet, a metabolic defect, or diuretic medications.

Water Therapy

To slow and prevent the crystallization of uric acid, drink 2 quarts of water a day. For pain, apply hot compresses to the afflicted joint, or bathe the joint in hot water.

General Therapy

One can lower uric acid levels by eating cherries, blueberries, or other dark red or blue berries every day. Folic acid, part of the B-complex family of nutrients, inhibits the production of uric acid, and vitamin C is valuable because it expedites excretion of uric acid. Other forms of prevention include eating a low-fat, high-fiber diet and watching one's weight, because obesity aggravates gout symptoms. Avoid these foods, which trigger attacks: organ meats, sardines, anchovies, dried peas, lentils, and other legumes. Alcoholic beverages, particularly red wine and beer, can also precipitate an attack, as can a niacin (B_3) or vitamin A supplement. Avoid fructose, an ingredient in many soft drinks and jellies. For pain, herbalists recommend an application of Balm of Gilead ointment. An experienced acupuncturist can lessen the pain of a gout attack.

GUM PROBLEMS

Water Therapy

Brush the teeth at least twice a day to avoid letting the mouth become a breeding ground for bacteria. Use a soft toothbrush.

Use any high-pressure irrigation device such as a Water-Pik to root out food caught between the teeth.

Release 3 to 4 drops of the Australian antiseptic tea tree oil into a glass of water, and swish it as a mouthwash. Most people have excellent results in several months.

The ancient Egyptians used myrrh for all sorts of antiseptic needs. Today we find myrrh has a particular affinity for the mouth. Add a few drops of myrrh to 2 tablespoons of water. Goldenseal powder is often combined with tincture of myrrh and is an excellent addition to any mouthwash for spongy gums.

Use the following herbs as table teas after meals: sage, chamomile, stinging nettle, and peppermint.

HAY FEVER

Water Therapy

Well before the expected hay fever season starts, each morning and evening whiff and expel a salt-water solution through each nostril. This cleanses the nasal passages and leaves them better prepared to resist pollen attacks.

Prior to and during the hayflower season, drink several glasses a day of the ancient Greek mixture "oxymel," made up of 1 teaspoon to 1 tablespoon each of apple cider vinegar and honey in a glass of water. This refreshing drink replaces many needed minerals, and sometimes is the only remedy needed by some hay fever sufferers.

Each day, drink copious amounts of water. In the early part of the morning, swallow a freeze-dried capsule of stinging nettle leaf. According to Dr. Andrew Weil, who lives in southern Arizona, an area rife with allergic rhinitis, freeze-dried nettle protects his patients and himself, and usually vanquishes the need to take antihistamines. Call 1-800-332-4372 for a product source.

During the Hayflower Season: Shower often to remove pollutants and pollen.

To clear sinus passages each day drink up to 2 quarts of cleansing liquids such as water or unsalted freshly juiced vegetables. Take freeze-dried capsules of nettle leaf. Inhale steam from a room vaporizer, a boiling pot of water, or a steamy bathroom to thin mucus and ease its expulsion from clogged sinuses.

To ease the pain from a sinus attack, apply hot moist cloths or a half-filled hot water bottle to the area of the cheekbones and eyes. Occasionally during the week, utilize these foot applications: hot leg baths alternated with hot and cold footbaths. Congestion in the nasal area will be controlled and may even disappear with occasional application of wet stocking therapy during sleep hours.

During the height of the attacks keep toning digestive organs with daytime applications of the cold abdomen compress technique. Renew the compress every 3 hours.

Each day drink 2 cups of either red clover or fenugreek tea.

In France, country people remedy hay fever attacks by combining 1 cup of scalded milk with 1 tablespoon of grated onion; drink the preparation while it is warm.

General Therapy

The following are strategies for preventing and overcoming hay fever situations: Purchase air conditioners, which can help to keep pollen out of the home, car, and workplace. HEPA air purifiers will help control microorganisms and microparticles in the air and will eliminate extraneous vapors, smells, and harmful volatile compounds. Check in the Yellow Pages for HEPA sources.

Whenever you participate in an outdoor activity, remember to remove pollen from the clothes and hair by changing clothes and showering out the pollen. Also, keep in mind that pollen migrates indoors on the fur of pets. Make the tough decision to keep a pet either outdoors or indoors.

A variety of vitamin supplements can boost the immune system and make it more resistant to allergic reactions. Dr. Andrew Weil advises taking doses of 400 mg of quercetin, a supplement active in preventing hay fever, twice a day between meals for two weeks prior to an expected hay fever attack, as well as throughout the allergic season. Do not take if pregnant. In addition, eat vitamin C rich foods, especially the inner flesh of citrus peel containing bioflavonoids, a substance which helps prevent clogging of nasal passages. Cut organic orange or lemon peel strips, soak them in apple cider vinegar and honey and then add the combination to herbal tea drinks. Garlic cloves or garlic capsules can help relieve head congestion. Other invaluable nutritional supplements in addition to vitamin C and bioflavonoids are vitamin A, vitamin E, vitamin B complex (including vitamins B_5 and B_6), coenzyme Q10, proteolytic enzymes, zinc, calcium, magnesium, manganese, pycnogenol, and kelp. Avoid drinking alcohol during the pollen season as alcohol causes blood vessels in the nose to swell, creating congestion. Consider the advantages of acupuncture treatments: studies show that patients feel better, more energized, warmer, and more relaxed after such procedures.

HEADACHES

Headaches can be symptoms of an internal problem, or they can be caused by controllable outside forces. It is not only useful but imperative to check and, when possible, eliminate the causal agents. Headaches that are generated from within the body may be due to digestive problems such as a sluggish liver, indigestion, constipation, or inflammation of the stomach; kidney or bowel problems; high blood pressure; or anemia. Outside factors include such diverse causes as sun glare, overheated or underventilated rooms, or tiny gas leaks from a heater, stove, or dryer. There are three types of headaches: functional, organic, and circulatory.

HEADACHES

Causes	Therapy
	Functional Headaches

Acute toxic headache
  Drug poisoning
  Infection
  Acute nephritis
  Uremia
	Institute immediate and vigorous treatment of causative factors.
	
	Relieve congestion with ice bags to carotid arteries and base of head.

Chronic toxic headache
  Rheumatism
  Arthritis
  Gout
  Sluggish liver
	Finding the causative factor is important. Water measures should be tonic and elminative, but may take weeks or months to overcome the problem, since it is chronic.
	
	Wrap calf of the leg from ankle to knee in single folded cloth dipped in fuller's earth and water. It can remain on for several hours. Blood is taken from the head and ache disappears.
	
	Alternate hot and cold compresses to head are generally soothing. Single cold compresses will also be helpful.
	
	Go outdoors, walk, sit in sunshine during early morning or late afternoon, but always be careful of overexposure.
	
	Investigate pressure therapy, manipulative therapy. Massage head frequently.

Migraine	This problem only responds to long-range tonic and eliminative water therapy. Check into reflex points of liver, stomach, and pelvis, and concentrate shower stream on these points.

continued on next page

Causes	Therapy

Working outdoors may be helpful.

Organic Headaches

Meningitis	Water therapy is not totally satisfactory here because of the intracranial pressure.
	Use methods to divert the head congestion.

Circulatory Headaches

Anemia	Alternate hot and cold compresses to head. Repeat daily, or on alternate days.
	Apply cold friction massage to body. Both of these stimulate circulation.
Too much congestion (hyperemic)	Deplete blood supply with either:

1. Fan shower to feet for 1 minute. Massage neck and shoulders and rest.
2. Hot footbaths, ice bags to carotid arteries (large arteries of neck).

Either of these tend to give relief.

Congestion due to toxemia or from studying too hard, or concentrating too hard	Use either alternate hot and cold leg bath or alternate hot and cold percussion shower to feet.
Passive congestion (as from a cold)	Same as for anemia—alternate hot and cold compress to head. Follow with hot footbath or hot leg pack. Finish with cold friction massage or cold percussion shower to feet.
	The brain is very sensitive to over-congestion. Therefore, applications to the feet ending with cold overcome the passive congestion, and keep the blood flow away from the head.

Water Therapy

When I am working hard on any project that requires sustained energy and clear thinking. I frequently walk in a half-bath of cold water for a few minutes, or sit in the cold bathwater for a few seconds. Both these techniques relieve brain fatigue.

Reflex Points for Head: Use short cold-water applications to hands, head, or feet. Short cold showers or brief cold shallow sit baths are also helpful.

HEART PROBLEMS

The objective of water therapy in acute heart problems is to sustain vital activity and to stimulate the heart by either reflex or direct action. Many physicians feel that some heart problems are due to reflex action from the stomach, and urge that this area receive exceptional attention.

Always consult a physician for any heart troubles. You may use water therapy as secondary therapy for heart problems. Also read the latest information on how nutrition and meditation can help to reverse some forms of heart disease. Use the following cold-water therapy as a secondary therapy—it can be a remarkable backup.

Water Therapy

The ice bag is one of the most efficient tonics for the heart. Cold friction-massage treatment, however, has the greatest range of use in treating organic heart problems. It can be used from the initial acute stage all through the recovery period. A prolonged, fan, no-pressure, neutral shower over the heart slows the heartbeat and strengthens the organ. Slapping the chest with a cold towel increases heart rate and force.

If no physician or emergency medical treatment is available, use CPR. The following water treatments are stimulating.

ACUTE SHOCK

If no professional help is available:

1. Place a hot moist compress on the heart for 2 minutes. Dry gently.

How to Use Water as a Secondary Treatment for the Heart

Tonic Water Treatments	Why/How Used
Cold friction massage	Greatest range of use in organic heart problems. Can be used in the initial stage to recovery period.
Ice bag treatments	Efficient tonic for the heart. According to clinical studies in hydrotherapy, when ice is placed over the heart, indications of collapse rapidly disappear.
Slap chest with cold towel. Apply prolonged, fan-shaped, no pressure, neutral-temperature shower to the heart area.	To increase heart rate and force. To slow heartbeat. To strengthen the heart.

2. Massage the area with ice for 30 seconds. Dry gently. (If ice is not available, at each inhalation of breath, gently slap the chest with a cold, wet towel. Repeat these steps 3 to 4 times.
3. After repetition, vigorously massage the heart area.
4. Alternate immediately with a cold compress for 5 minutes.

ANGINA

Try these in addition to traditional remedies.

Pain Relief: Plunge the hands into a hot hand bath for 15 seconds, or plunge the feet into a hot footbath for 15 seconds. Repeat every 5 minutes until there is an improvement. The water can be extremely hot.

General Therapy: Apply a hot moist compress over the heart area for 1 minute. Alternate immediately with a cold compress for 5 minutes.

Old Czech Country Remedy for "Heart Cramps": This is said to relieve both heart and asthma spasms without any side effects. In advance, put aside and label "Save for Emergency":

- 1 gallon old fermented apple cider
- 1 ounce or more melissa or lemon balm tea or flaxseed oil

In two different nonaluminum pots, heat up about a half-gallon of the fermented cider and 1 ounce of the flaxseed oil or melissa tea. Heat the cider to a fast boil. Remove from the heat. Dip two large hand towels in the hot liquid, wring out, and place as hot as possible on both arms at once. The hot fruit acid relieves the cramps. At the same time dip a folded washcloth into the hot flaxseed oil or melissa tea and apply to the heart area.

MYOCARDITIS

Cold has an inhibitory effect on the motor-stimulating nerves. Clinical studies in hydrotherapy show that an ice pack placed over the heart many brief times during the day, for 3 to 6 days, allows the inflamed area to recover.

ACUTE ENDOCARDITIS

For problems associated with rheumatic fever, in the initial stage of inflammation, do the following:

1. Renew cold compresses to the heart every 15 minutes.
2. Three times a day, apply moderate-strength cold-water friction massage to each part of the body. Start with one arm, keeping the rest of the body covered with a large towel. Go to the next arm, then massage the chest, and so on.

When the inflammation is reduced:

1. Continue with the above cold friction massage and lightly massage the entire body.
2. Four to five times a day apply an ice bag to the heart for 20 to 30 minutes.

Before lunch, apply any of these tonic water therapies: cold friction massage, cold towel rub, hot footbath, hot moist compresses to the spine, jet showers or alternate hot and cold showers directed to the spinal area.

Two hours after lunch or two hours after supper, use alternate hot and cold footbaths. Always end with cold.

EDEMA

Edema is swelling of the ankles and/or limbs due to heart problems. Take alternate hot-water and cold-water ankle and leg baths, repeated 10 times. Make sure the water completely covers the swollen ankle(s) or limb(s).

Footbaths: Dip swollen feet in a hot-water footbath for 1 to 2 minutes. Immediately alternate with a cold-water footbath for 10 to 15 seconds. Friction-dry with a towel after each cold immersion. Start the cold immersions with normal tap water, and gradually increase the cold with ice cubes. If only the ankle (and not the limb) is swollen, massage the entire area when the sequence of alternate hot and cold is finished.

HEAT REACTIONS

HEAT EXHAUSTION

Prevention

During hot spells it is extremely important to drink copious amounts of liquids, especially water. Avoid drinking alcohol and caffeine, which act as diuretics and increase the body's need for liquid.

As often as possible during a hot day, hold the wrists and ankles under cold running water.

Apply frequent cold, wet compresses to the back of the neck.

Eat watermelon.

Heat Exhaustion Signals

During excessively hot weather pay attention to body signals such as dizziness, chills, nausea, headache, fuzzy thinking, and clamminess. If you feel any of these symptoms, get out of the heat as quickly as possible. Be aware that the following medications influence one's ability to cope with the heat: laxatives, appetite suppressants, diuretics, sedatives, antihistamines, some thyroid hormones, and Parkinson's disease drugs.

What to Do—Water Therapy

LCD—Lie down, Cool off, Drink water and other liquids.

Have the heat-exhausted person lie down with the feet elevated and the head lower than the feet. Immediately cool the person with wet cloths to the head and body. If possible, put large, wet towels on the trunk of the body. If you can, give the person an instant cool bath. If such a bath isn't possible, do everything possible to cool the person further—use cold, wet washcloths to cool the armpits, groin, neck, and wrist.

Have the person sip cold (not iced) drinks that contain ⅛ teaspoon of salt, which replaces missing minerals (electrolytes) washed out with the intense perspiration loss. Fruit juice, tomato juice, lemonade, peppermint tea, and ginseng tea are also effective drinks. Avoid caffeine and caffeine-laced drinks, which increase the body's need for liquids.

Follow our tropical and subtropical neighbors and add a small pinch or two of cayenne pepper powder to foods or to the above drinks to stimulate and restore the entire system.

General Therapy

There are two excellent Chinese trigger points for heatstroke and sunstroke: For several seconds, press the bony part of the web between the thumb and the index finger, release, and repeat. This is the famed Ho Ku point, useful for headaches and diarrhea as well as constipation. Also press and release the middle area under the nostrils and over the lips. Two cell (tissue) salts are useful for a strong reaction to heat. Take 5 natrum mur. 6x. Fifteen minutes later alternate with 5 tablets of ferrum phos. 6x. This can be repeated up to 5 times during the day.

HEAT RASH OR PRICKLY HEAT

Babies have not yet fully developed their ability to sweat and tend to get little heat pimples called prickly heat or heat rash. In hot weather make sure that the baby is drinking some water and is not dehydrated. A child who is even slightly dehydrated becomes more sensitive to heat. Adults also get prickly heat reactions, especially between the thighs, under the armpits, and under the breasts.

Prevention

Keep children (and adults) out of the sun as much as possible. For babies: Change diapers often, and avoid all plastic, even plastic changing pads. Use cornstarch to dust the baby after changing the diapers. "Air dry" the baby as much as possible. Avoid tight clothes that chafe and synthetic fabrics that don't breathe.

Water Therapy

Place the child in a series of cool to tepid baths. If the child is old enough, a series of cool showers will be refreshing. Dust off the child with a small amount of cornstarch. One of the following three substances in a bath will relieve itching and promote wellness:

1. Use up to 1 cup of Aveeno colloidal oatmeal in the bathwater.
2. Add a quarter of a cup of apple cider vinegar to the bathwater for a child, and a full cup of apple cider vinegar for an adult. The skin should be encased in a high pH acid cover. Apple cider vinegar restores this acid mantle.
3. Apply some baking soda directly to the rash to help relieve the itching. Also add several tablespoons of baking soda to the bathwater.

HEMORRHOIDS

Water Therapy

Constipation is the chief cause of hemorrhoids. Use water and fiber to overcome constipation.

Start each day by drinking 2 glasses of cold water. This encourages peristalsis, wavelike muscular contractions of the alimentary canal, which help overcome constipation.

During the day, drink at least 6 to 8 glasses of water. In general also drink herb teas and juice.

For Pain: To reduce inflammation, apply absorbent cotton pads soaked in either witch hazel extract plus water, or strong chamomile tea.

Both wet heat and ice applications work well in alleviating hemorrhoid pain. These hot and/or cold procedures may be alternated as needed.

Use heat to overcome spasms. Although the warm shallow (sitz) baths reduce itching and help shrink swollen rectal veins and inflammation, the hot shallow sitz bath (or if a bath is not available, hot moist compresses) is the most effective relief for spasms. When taking these shallow baths, place 6 to 8 inches of warm water in the tub and sit with the feet elevated on a rubber pillow or leaning against the sides of the tub. When rectal itching is also a problem, add a half-cup of colloidal oatmeal (Aveeno) to the bathwater. This type of oatmeal dissolves easily in water. If it is not available, grind regular oatmeal into tiny particles and use in the bathwater. Neutral or warm bidet upward showers, which can be installed in the toilet, are also helpful. Hot footbaths may also be employed to draw congestion away from the anal area.

Ice-cold procedures are very soothing. The following applications should be made-up in advance so that they can be used instantly. Prepare a series of cotton makeup pads soaked in witch hazel or chamomile tea. Wring out. Put each one into a sandwich-sized plastic bag, and lay the group of plastic bags flat on a piece of cardboard in the freezer. When needed, apply frozen, one at a time.

Add boiling-hot water to 2 tablespoons of crushed sage seeds. Steep and discard the seeds. Place a soft cotton pad in the water, wring out, and apply either hot or cold to the painful area.

General Therapy

Take vitamin C and vitamin E supplements. Add more fiber to the diet, including whole-grain breads and cereals, and many green vegetables and fruits each day. A high-fiber diet with plenty of liquids is likely to prevent the formation of hemorrhoids and make the stools bulkier and softer, thus causing less straining. Try eating around the same time each day. Chew food slowly and thoroughly. Never ignore an urge to defecate. Include some brisk walking and other exercise in your daily routine. Learn to breathe in an easy way, especially when lifting, stooping, and squatting.

HERPES SIMPLEX

Water Therapy

Most patients feel tingling, burning, stinging, or tightness on the site of a prior infection, which may occur minutes or hours before the actual blister forms. Pay attention to this prodrome (warning), for there is a water therapy that can stop it in its tracks. Immediately massage ice on the area of tightness—a few minutes on, a few minutes off, and repeat again and again. If you get to the site in time, the ice massage will stop the blister from forming.

General Therapy

Purchase a glycyrrhizinic acid ointment, made of licorice root, which is known to inhibit herpes simplex growth. Apply as an alternate to the early ice massage before the blister emerges, or if it does emerge, apply several times a day to the sores. Another beneficial ointment contains zinc sulphate 0.025. Some practitioners combine this ointment with an 8 percent lithium succinate solution to produce a substance that can disrupt virus reproduction. Apply this after breakfast, lunch, and dinner. Vitamin E directly from a capsule can be applied to a dried blister to accelerate healing. Herpes outbreaks emerge during stress periods, so it is imperative to maintain a strong, efficient immune system. To ward off attacks, avoid stressful situations and eat an optimum diet, especially foods containing the antiviral amino acid lysine. Foods that are high in lysine are salmon, halibut, brewer's yeast, and sardines. Avoid any food that contains arginine, a lysine-antagonist and a trigger for many herpes attacks. Key arginine foods to avoid are chocolate, peanuts, and most nuts, especially almonds, Brazil nuts, cashews, pecans, and walnuts. Boost the immune system with 2,000 mg of ester vitamin C; echinacea in capsule, spray, or tincture; a multivitamin with a high dose of beta carotene; 15 mg of zinc to inhibit herpes simplex duplication within the body; and vitamin E taken internally to shorten the duration of the eruptions and expedite internal healing.

HICCUPS

Water Therapy

The world abounds in easy and effective hiccup remedies. Each works by shocking the diaphragm, glottis, or vagus or phrenic nerves.

Hiccups will usually stop after you drink water. Sometimes several glasses of water are needed. One water routine passed down through the centuries consists of stretching the neck out to drink the water on the farthest side of the glass.

Pineapple juice, or any acidic juice, is a great hiccup remedy.

HIGH BLOOD PRESSURE

Water Therapy

There are three excellent water therapies that reduce high blood pressure:

1. Reduce internal pressure with a neutral-temperature enema.
2. Induce sweating with hot baths or a sauna. Use a cold compress on the head.
3. Reduce a high blood pressure headache by diverting blood from the head to the feet. To accomplish this, immerse the feet in a hot mustard powder footbath or apply alternate hot and cold streams of water to the feet. Sebastian Kneipp, one of the great codifiers of hydrotherapy, recommends wrapping the calves with a clay-dipped cloth for two hours. Dip a long strip of cloth or a soft Ace bandage into a gruel-like solution of neutral clay and water. Wrap each calf from the ankle to the knee. If there is any unusual reaction, such as palpitations, discontinue immediately.

General Therapy

Fifty million Americans, most over 60 years of age, suffer from high blood pressure. Common symptoms are headaches, dizziness, ringing in the ears, tingling in the hands and feet, blurred vision, palpitations, nosebleeds, drowsiness, and confusion. Changes in lifestyle and diet include a low-fat and high-fiber diet abundant in antioxidant supplements. Avoid red meats, increase fruits and vegetables in the diet, and use olive oil, a monounsaturated fat. Some complementary physicians believe that the primary cause of most high blood pressure is a food allergy, so this should be investigated.

According to cardiologist Dr. Stephen Sinatra, author of *Heartbreak and Heart Disease*, about 35 percent of high blood pressure patients may have a coenzyme Q10 deficiency, a substance, he says, that functions like a vitamin as it rescues body tissues that have been damaged by free radicals. Dr. Sinatra starts his patients on 30 mg and works up to 90 mg twice a day for one to three months. Foods containing this substance are sardines, salmon, and mackerel.

Other foods that help control high blood pressure are celery stalks or juice, bananas and oranges (which are high in potassium), green leafy vegetables and vegetable juices, foods high in essential fatty acids (as well as capsules of Max EPA, borage oil, or black currant seed oil), and garlic. Use hawthorn berry extract to strengthen the heart, and a natural diuretic such as corn silk tea or parsley, or asparagus, or watermelon. Each day for a month, eat a handful of sunflower seeds. Avoid foods high in salt, which is often concealed in such foods as canned soup and vegetables, diet sodas, soy sauce, softened water, pickles, olives, ham, and bacon. Also avoid smoked and aged cheeses, animal fats, gravies, and coffee, because caffeine can temporarily raise blood pressure. Some susceptible people increase their blood pressure by eating sugar and processed foods containing sugar.

Acupuncture treatments often show dramatic results by rebalancing the body and restoring function. Exercise at least three times a week, and practice yoga and yoga breathing. Take massage treatments. Stop smoking. Watch out for any side effects from prescription drugs.

HERNIA (HIATUS HERNIA)

Water Therapy

Here is a water therapy tip that may help you. One man who sometimes pops his hiatus hernia tells me that drinking a glass of warm water and jumping up and down fixes the problem right away.

INCONTINENCE

A common and daunting problem is the involuntary loss of fluid when sneezing, coughing, laughing, or lifting objects. This frequently happens to women when the pelvic floor muscles become weakened by pregnancy, childbirth, and menopause. Water therapies are important remedies for the problem of incontinence.

Water Therapy

Drink copious amounts of water to flush the urinary tract of bacteria. If you suffer from nighttime incontinence, drink water mainly in the morning and taper off your intake in the afternoon.

Cold-water treatments are known to build up resistance and immunity and are an integral part of European treatments of incontinence, which involve progressively longer cold-water "treading," or walking in cold water. First, stream cold water over the big toe for seconds, or if possible, minutes. The next day and for the following days, place all the toes under the cold running water, and as soon as possible include the entire foot. Do this every day, slowly increasing the amount of cold water, until you can fill a bathtub with several inches of cold water and walk around in it without discomfort. Soon, it will actually feel pleasurable. Eventually, you should be able to walk (tread) in cold water up to the calves of the legs. Hold on to a safety bar while marching in the water. Patients with heart or circulation problems should avoid this exercise.

General Therapy

A professional shiatsu massage can often improve incontinence. Minimize your intake of coffee, tea, and other caffeinated beverages. Decrease your consumption of foods with sugar and refined carbohydrates in order to avoid a buildup of yeast and bacteria.

Herbal Aids: Three safe herbs are used in Europe for incontinence or bed-wetting. Capsules and/or tincture of St. John's wort act on the nervous system to control bedwetting. Try 2 to 30 drops of gentian tincture in water at midday or evening. Or try sweet sumac, a North American plant that most herbalists use specifically for bedwetting: 5 to 10 drops in water 2 times a day. Hyperforat (Klien), Suburgen (Vogel & Weber), and Nierenklar (Salus) are effective German products that can be ordered through your pharmacy or health food store.

Kegel Exercises: The most important thing you can do to fight incontinence is to learn Kegel exercises, which strengthen the bladder and bowel muscles. The pelvic floor muscles are alternately tightened and relaxed during urination by starting and stopping the flow of water and by tightening and relaxing the muscles of the rectum as if trying to stop a stool from being passed. Since these are "invisible" exercises, they can be done throughout the day while standing or sitting. In the rare instance that a woman cannot do these exercises on her own, three other professional medical approaches can be utilized: inserting progressively larger cone-shaped weights into the vagina, biofeedback sessions, or electrical stimulation. Men with incontinence can take biofeedback sessions.

PELVIC FLOOR KEGEL EXERCISES FOR INCONTINENCE

These exercises can be done unobtrusively when alone, and can be done all through the day. Doing these exercises lessens the chance of involuntarily passing urine, having a uterine prolapse, and developing backaches. Another advantage is that they enhance sexual pleasure.

To strengthen the pubococcygeus muscle, do these exercises for several minutes every day. Start with two or more repeated sessions and build up, or do two sessions with 20 to 25 repeats. The final results will be well worth the effort.

On the toilet	Stop and start the flow of urine and pull up (contract) the vagina.
	Tighten and relax the muscles of the rectum as if stopping a stool from passing.
Sitting, standing	Tightly contract the same muscle that controls the flow of urine. Hold for 2 seconds. Relax for 2 seconds. Repeat. The goal is to be able to hold for 10 seconds.
	Contract the rectal muscles as if stopping a stool, for a count of 2. Work up to a count of 10.
Lying on your back on the floor	Bend the knees so that the feet rest on the floor. Relax. Using a short upward movement, raise, lower, and squeeze the pelvic area. If you have trouble with this exercise, take a series of yoga classes to learn it.
Using internal weights	Your physician can supply you with cone-shaped, progressively increased, internal weights for the vagina. These weights, which are effective for stress incontinence, are also available via some mail-order catalogs.
Biofeedback	The results from biofeedback are said to be excellent. Ask your gynecologist for a referral.
Electrical stimulation	Very successful. Ask your physician for a referral to a gynecologist.

INDIGESTION

ACUTE INDIGESTION

Water Therapy

On a general basis, hydrate the cells and the entire system by drinking about 2 quarts of water each day.

During an acute attack of indigestion, it often helps to vomit. Drinking warm water acts as an emetic. If this doesn't work, add a few grains of mustard powder to the warm water. It should cause vomiting. Afterwards, drink additional warm water to cleanse the stomach and dilute the acids of decomposition.

Peppermint tea has always been used to soothe the stomach. Other good teas to quiet the digestive system are chamomile, fennel, and melissa (lemon balm). Melisana, the German Carmelite formula, can also instantly soothe stomach upsets.

A chamomile enema soothes and quiets the colon. A coffee enema can be used to detoxify and cleanse the colon area, but is very powerful and should be used cautiously.

If you are on the verge of vomiting, but would prefer not to do so, apply an ice bag over the stomach and a hot water bottle on the vertebrae between the shoulders. This should control the urge to heave.

To prevent attacks, take chamomile or peppermint tea. On trips away from home, carry peppermint tea bags or vials of peppermint spirit and add a few drops to just-boiled water. Drink it as a soothing tea and to relieve spasms.

Whenever possible, wear the cold double abdominal compress. This works both for acute attacks and as a long-range strengthener for the digestive organs. It has a general heating effect, which is also very comforting. If you sense that you are going to have trouble with digestion, fast for a day or two on pure bottled water, distilled water, or organic apples or apple juice.

FLATULENCE

Gently press the seeds of fennel, caraway, or anise between the fingers to release the volatile oil. Pour boiling water on the seeds, steep and discard seeds, and then drink the tea. An easy shortcut is to pour a few drops of anisette (aniseed liqueur) into hot water or another digestive tea.

Add a pinch of cayenne pepper to any of the above digestive teas or to boiling-hot water to help regulate the digestive system.

PAIN

For abdominal cramps from indigestion, take a 10- to 15-minute hot shower until the stomach area turns bright red. If a shower is not available, apply hot compresses to the abdomen every 10 minutes until there is some relief. Poultices containing chopped raw onion or raw cabbage may also be applied to bring comfort to the area.

CHRONIC INDIGESTION

As a preventive measure, take tea with 1 teaspoon of slippery elm bark powder before meals. A small amount of honey may be added to this tea.

General Therapy

It is always beneficial to engage in deep, relaxed, conscious breathing to assuage gastrointestinal pain. For a burning, acid stomach, the late Swiss naturopath Amos Vogel advised chewing some dry rolled oats to neutralize the acid and help the pains to subside. Potato broth, steamed parsnips, papaya, or cooked carrots are calming foods to eat. Avoid overeating fatty foods. Eat lots of papaya and pineapple, both of which contain digestive enzymes that break down proteins. Avoid citrus foods when you have indigestion. However, raw vegetable juices such as carrots, celery, and greens may help, as do blackberry and organic apple juices. Cleansing the entire digestive tract with a professional colonic may prove to be a lifestyle turnaround. Also try reducing your food intake one day a week. Some people even practice "Monday juice and/or water fasts" as a general principle for staying healthy and to cleanse and quiet the digestive system. If none of these things work, check out the possibility of a sensitivity to one or more foods.

CHRONIC INDIGESTION

Water therapy is an adjunct to good diet, careful chewing of foods, and exercise. The proper sequence of water therapy can greatly increase the tone of the body and the capacity of the body to digest and absorb nutrients.

Water Therapy

In general, take frequent showers, starting with a few seconds of a gentle neutral stream and concluding with a few seconds of a neutral jet stream. Direct the showers to the upper middle stomach and to the area slightly below.

On Arising: One hour before the morning meal, sip a glass of lukewarm water. Or, if you produce an excess of hydrochloric acid, drink hot water on arising. Flex knees and vigorously massage abdomen for 5 minutes, or until gurgling is heard and the water passes from the stomach into the intestines.

After drinking the water, take a 10-minute neutral bath (95°F to 98°F). Conclude bath with tonic friction sponging, sectional cold mitten rub, or cold shower.

In the Evening: Several hours after the evening meal, and before going to bed, apply a cold double abdominal compress. In the morning, wash the abdomen with cold water. The compress relieves congested conditions throughout the alimentary canal by drawing blood to the surface.

INFECTION

The natural traditional approach to treating infection or abscesses is threefold. Kill the infection with as many natural substances as possible; build up immediate and long-term resistance through the use of nutrients such vitamins C, A, and E and essential fatty acids, quercetin, and zinc; and plan long-range strategies such as avoiding areas of contamination in living and working areas. These strategies include removing dust and dust mites from the house, preventing furnace dust from blowing into the house, cleaning air conditioners regularly, vacuuming often, and cleansing humidifiers. If infections happen often, act like a detective and track down possible sources.

Water Therapy

When bacteria and viruses were first discovered, we learned to scrub our hands several times a day. Nowadays we've forgotten the advantages of this simple procedure. Wash your hands often, especially if you are in contact with someone who has a contagious infection. It also helps to always wash your hands after returning home from work or school, after a bus ride, after going to the movies, and especially during a cold or flu epidemic. Teachers and parents should instruct children to wash their hands after playtime, before eating, and upon arriving home. This little gesture will cut down on lots of cold misery.

Soap now comes in easily dispensed liquid form. Control the home and office environments by scrubbing everyday objects such as water cooler handles, light switches, doorknobs, telephone handles and mouthpieces, refrigerator door handles, and coffee or tea pots.

Dentures are sometimes at the root of puzzling recurrent infections, especially infections of the throat, nose, and face. The medical journal *The Lancet* advises us that some facial infections can be overcome by simply not wearing dentures for a few days. The way to clean dentures is to soak them in a cleaning solution to which some bleach has been added, followed by a toothbrushing rinse.

General Therapy

Natural antibiotics include a variety of culinary herbs, plants, medicinal oils, and foods. Garlic, which can be used raw in salads and other foods, has the ability to combat gram-negative infections. Horseradish, which will smite many bacteria, can be made into a pungent sauce useful with many foods, including one famously identified with brisket of beef. Honey is another amazing natural antibiotic, which has been used since ancient Egyptian times to kill bacteria in wounds. Because it is so sweet, it is an easy addition to tart lemonade, which has its own ability to cleanse the body, and to such anti-infection plants as rosemary, lavender, sage, rue, wormwood, and mint. Echinacea or purple coneflower, a plant the American Plains Indians discovered, is now a part of many people's daily regimen to combat colds and flu. Vitamin C and zinc are also effective immune boosters. Eat citrus foods for the C content, and egg yolks, fish, whole grains, and tofu for zinc.

INFLAMMATION

General Therapy

Vitamin C has strong anti-inflammatory properties. Take high doses of vitamin C supplements. Eat and drink citrus fruits. Omega-3 fatty acids in the form of fish oil can be taken for any internal inflammation. To reduce digestive inflammation, take capsules of the anti-inflammatory herb turmeric, and reduce gastritis inflammation with daily chlorophyll tablets. Many herbs are extremely beneficial in reducing inflammation. Calendula ointment can be slathered on most skin inflammation. Marshmallow root tea and compresses have been used for centuries to heal internal inflammation. Clean, unsprayed plantain leaves, even those from local parks, are excellent "Band-Aids" for external inflammation, including tough-to-heal finger inflammations. When there are no skin cuts, arnica ointment can reduce pain quickly.

MINOR INFLAMMATION

Water Therapy

Early Stage of Inflammation—Ice: Prolonged cold-water applications are effective in treating minor inflammations. Apply an ice bag or frozen ice pack over the inflammation for 20 minutes of every hour. For joints that are inflamed but not hot, use contrast hot and cold therapy to soothe the pain by alternating applications of an ice pack and a hot water bottle.

Another prolonged ice application that actually heats up from within the body is the homemade "frozen bandage." To make such bandages, take three soft washcloths. Dip each in cold water. Wring out. Fold in half. Place each washcloth in a plastic sandwich bag. Stack the plastic-encased washcloths on flat cardboard and place flat in the freezer. When a spasm or an inflammation hits, apply the frozen bandage to it. The body will rush blood and heat to the area, and the cold, frozen cloth will soon become warm and pliable. When this occurs, apply fresh frozen bandages, in a series of two or three. The result is usually quite spectacular.

To fight urinary or joint inflammation, drink a cup of fresh celery juice.

Bumps, bruises, and other minor inflammations can be reduced by applying witch hazel compresses.

Later Stages of Inflammation—Moist Heat: During the latter stage of an inflammation use hot, moist heat applications such as compresses, partial baths, or tepid or neutral-temperature water jet showers on the inflamed parts.

If there is no throbbing pain, immerse the inflamed area in alternate hot and cold partial baths.

INTERNAL DEEP INFLAMMATION

Water Therapy

For inflammation in soft tissues, use cold applications. For inflammation on bony sections, use hot applications; for instance, at the mastoid bone behind each ear.

MASTOIDITIS

Use only heat. Even the slightest cold application increases the pain.

ABSCESS

Apply a hot, moist compress over the inflammation. Heat alone relieves the pain, but the action doesn't last long. Therefore, also apply an ice bag over the large artery supplying blood to the abscessed area.

EYE INFLAMMATION

Use a cold compress.

FACE INFLAMMATION

Spray with cold water or apply a cold compress.

ANUS, SCROTUM, PROSTATE, HEMORRHOID INFLAMMATIONS

Renew a cold compress every 15 minutes. At night use a T-shaped genital or hemorrhoid compress.

PLEURISY

Use only heat.

INFLAMMATIONS IN CHILDREN

To reduce internal heat, give the child a spoonful of cold water every half-hour and 1 teaspoon of cold-pressed vegetable oil once a day.

Apply a cold-water compress that has been folded into thirds or a single cold-water and apple cider vinegar compress to the inflamed area every half-hour. Quick "dunks" in and out of cold water up to the armpits several times a day will accelerate healing.

If a child has a finger inflammation, treat the entire body. Friction-rub the entire body with a cold washcloth. Dry the child immediately.

See "Inflammation Chart" on pages 228–229.

INFLAMMATORY BOWEL DISEASE

Water Therapy

Drink at least 2 quarts of water a day to combat the fluids you may be losing from diarrhea. See "Diarrhea" section for foods to choose and those to avoid.

General Therapy

Inflammatory bowel disease (IBD) is linked to two other chronic digestive problems, Crohn's disease and ulcerative colitis. There are no known cures for these diseases, but there are some interesting natural approaches that may help. Raspberry tea is rich in tannin, an astringent that fights nasty bacteria in the gut. Patients with inflammatory bowel disease should investigate a possible connection between the problem and food allergies, which can trigger attacks. For instance, it is imperative to observe the connection between IBD and wheat, sugar, eggs, citrus fruits, dairy products, and corn, even corn flakes, which many Crohn's disease and ulcerative colitis patients seem to consume. On the whole, dairy products are to be avoided although yogurt appears to be tolerated. Dr. Ronald Hoffman of New York advises his patients to stay away from meat, especially red meat, and suggests eating fiber, which he says, "helps whisk out bile acids, which can turn ulcerative colitis into colon cancer."

IBD patients with Crohn's disease or ulcerative colitis are usually put on a regimen of strong anti-inflammatories and/or strong antibiotics. Antibiotics will clean the gut of all bacteria, beneficial bacteria as well. This leaves patients at high risk for yeast infections. Compensate for the loss of friendly flora by taking capsules of a nondairy bioculture that contains potent amounts of acidophilus, bifidus, and other cultures. Many top nutrition counselors prescribe Commensal, made by New Millennium Foods (Sedna Specialty Health Products, Andrews, NC 28901) an expensive but formidable product with 15 billion viable culture cells per capsule.

INSECT BITES

Water Therapy

Getting stung by a wasp or bee is one of summer's less pleasant rites of passage; unfortunately, sometimes we get stung in the least pleasant of places, the mouth or throat, by an insect that has made its way into our sandwich or soda can. Gargle immediately with a solution of salt water—2 tablespoons of salt to a half-glass of water. To quicken the healing process and alleviate the pain, gargle with whey powder and apply one of these two compresses to the neck: a series of overlapping cabbage leaves that have been dipped into boiling-hot water, or a large clay pack. The clay pack can also be placed on the swollen area of the mouth.

IRRITABLE BOWEL SYNDROME

Water Therapy

Make a point of drinking at least 2 quarts of water a day to feed the cells and to avoid constipation.

For abdominal pain, take a hot sitz bath containing either apple cider vinegar or strong chamomile tea. Fill a bathtub with hot (100°F) water 6 to 8 inches deep and sit in it with your feet up on a pillow or on the sides of the tub. Add 1 cup of apple cider vinegar or chamomile tea to the bathwater.

INFLAMMATION CHART

For Inflammation or Congestion in This Area	Apply Water Here
Eye	Apply hot or cold to side of face or forehead. This dilates some of the terminal superficial branches of the carotids and depletes the deeper branches.
Pharynx and larynx	Apply a cold double compress to neck. This depletes the deeper organs and congests the surface vessels.
Pleurisy	Where congestion is limited, as in pleurisy, a hot moist compress can be used directly, as this dilates the posterior, lateral, and anterior cutaneous branches of the intercostal arteries, thereby withdrawing blood from the inflamed pleura.
Acute congestion	Hot double leg compress, or full hot blanket and cold compress or ice to affected lobe.
Kidney	Circulation in these organs decreased by hot application to the back, as this dilates the posterior branches of the lumbar and lower intercostal arteries. 1. Use hot moist compresses over the lower dorsal and lumbar spine for entire width of back. 2. Or use an ice bag on lower third of breastbone (sternum).
Stomach	Large applications centering at the middle lower abdomen and extending over the lower chest and sides of the abdomen.
Pelvic organs (bladder, uterus, ovaries, tubes, rectum, and prostate)	Acute: Start with hot vaginal douche. Use simultaneous water therapy: ice bag to groin and hot leg compress or hot leg compress and hip pack. Continue 20 to 30 minutes. Follow with cold mitten friction to the area. Repeat 2 to 3 times a day, if necessary.

continued on next page

For Inflammation or Congestion in This Area	Apply Water Here
	Chronic: Use hot sit bath, gradually lowering the temperature until it is quite cold. Stay in bath a few seconds to minutes. Use alternate hot and cold vaginal douche irrigation frequently. Also use tonic friction methods and alternate hot and cold showers to lower back, legs, and feet.
Spine (simple congestion)	Hot moist compresses to the spine. This diverts the blood to the arteries supplying the skin and muscles of the back from the spinal arteries.
Brain	1. Hot leg bath, with cold compress to head. 2. Hot moist compress to face, ears, and forehead (but not nose). Simultaneously apply ice bags to two carotid arteries at base of brain and top of head. 3. Compress to head and ice bags to carotid arteries.
Middle ear and mastoid	Apply very hot leg bath, hot moist cloths to mastoid bone, and simultaneous ice bag over carotid artery on same side as pain for 20 to 30 minutes. Follow with vigorous cold mitten friction massage to trunk and limbs.
Mastoiditis (inflammation of the mastoid bone)	Heat decreases pain of inflammation of bony areas. (Ice on the mastoid will increase pain.)

General Therapy

Check for food sensitivities, which vary from person to person. Eat small meals at frequent intervals. Avoid mealtime stresses, since these affect the digestive system. In general, eat little fat and avoid sugar, corn syrup, milk products, caffeine (also in drinks and over-the-counter medications), corn, wheat, MSG, nitrates, alcohol, carbonated beverages, and chewing gum. Get yourself checked for intestinal parasites. Avoid being deficient in unsaturated fatty acids. Eat yogurt to replenish friendly bacteria residing in the gut. Read up on yeast infections. Avoid beer and red wine, which can precipitate an attack. Valerian capsules are helpful for gastrointestinal spasms. Walking, swimming, and moderate bent-knee sit-ups are helpful to improve bowel muscle tone. Heal the irritated mucus lining of the digestive tract with mucilaginous marshmallow or slippery elm herbs. Alleviate discomfort with massage, reflexology, or shiatsu. Yoga, relaxation breathing, meditation, and biofeedback can help you manage the stress of this disease.

ITCHING

GENERAL ITCHING

Apply an ice bag to the area of the itching. Briefly immerse the itching part in very cold water. Apply a cold compress to relieve the itching.

Take a warm bath containing 1 or 2 cups of apple cider vinegar. Before taking the bath splash diluted apple cider vinegar over the itchy parts of the body. Apple cider vinegar restores the normal pH of the skin and will relieve some of the intense itchiness. This water healing is most useful for winter skin dryness and itchiness, insect bites, and sunburn itchiness. Compresses or splashes of apple cider vinegar combined with goldenseal will often relieve the extreme itch from poison ivy. Use 1 cup of the apple cider vinegar with 1 tablespoon of goldenseal powder or 10 drops of goldenseal tincture.

Use oatmeal, preferably the tiny particles of blended colloidal oatmeal Aveeno, as a backup for most itching ordeals, including hives, sunburn, and skin dryness. Place some as a wet mash directly on the itching part and wash it off later in a shower or bath, or use large amounts in a full bath. I have seen a child's hives disappear almost instantly after taking such a bath.

Splash witch hazel extract on insect bites, sunburn, and itching areas. Prepared extracts are available in most pharmacies. Purchase the Dickinson brand rather than the less expensive generic brands.

Drink ice water to numb the pain of itching from a heat rash.

RECTAL ITCHING

Rectal itching may be a warning of hemorrhoids, an indication of parasites within the intestinal tract, or too little hydrochloric acid in the stomach, a problem that occurs in many people after the age of 50. This acid, necessary for digestion, is easily replaced with tablets, usually buffered with the digestive enzyme betaine.

Pay particular attention to the cleanliness of the anal area. After each bowel movement clean the anus with a white facial tissue or cloth soaked with water and a neutral soap. Dry the area with still another facial tissue. Wash this area several times a day. Often it is helpful to apply a neutral, healing ointment such as zinc oxide.

General Therapy

The Lee Foundation for Nutritional Research issued a clinical report by Dr. N. Philip Norman on pruritus ani, intense chronic itching in the anal region. According to Dr. Norman many itching problems emanate from a buildup of internal toxicity. He suggests the following diet. Breakfast: fresh, uncooked fruit, such as berries, melon, unsulfured dried fruit; milk or buttermilk; and unsweetened coffee, coffee substitutes, or tea. Lunch: vegetable soup made without meat stock, or a raw or cooked vegetable salad, butter, and milk. Supper: a protein meal with no starch, such as vegetable soup that can contain some meat; meat or cheese, nuts or legumes; two cooked fresh vegetables; a large green salad; berries or melon for dessert; and unsweetened coffee, coffee substitute, or tea.

ITCHING IN CHILDREN

Most itching in children occurs during childhood diseases such as measles or chicken pox. Hives occur with various allergic reactions. All these conditions respond to baths with Aveeno, a colloidal oatmeal preparation. Scabies may affect the head. Sometimes a hot bath or shower produces mild to severe itching in adolescents with pityriasis rosea, which may show up on the face, hands, and feet.

A child with nonlocalized intense itching should be checked for possible liver malfunction, because itching can sometimes be caused by the accumulation of bile salts on the skin.

JET LAG

Water Therapy

Drink 1 glass of water for each hour in the air. This prevents dehydration and helps overcome the trauma of jet lag. A steward will supply you with bottled water on request. Do not drink alcoholic drinks while flying; they have twice the impact at air level that they do on the ground. Also avoid caffeine and sodas containing caffeine, which dehydrate the body.

Before the plane lands, splash your face with cold water and brush your teeth. This energizes and revives the entire system. If you are tired, fill the sink with cold water and plunge your hands into the water for a minute or so. Dry them vigorously.

General Therapy

Eat lightly on a flight, especially on long flights. Most airlines have banned smoking, and this is fortunate since smoking depletes the body's oxygen intake. To avoid further fluid retention and swelling during a flight, avoid high-sodium tomato juice and salted peanuts, as well as all other high-sodium snacks. Elevate the feet (your carry-on luggage will do) and each hour, take a stroll around the airplane. Airlines continue to save fuel by lessening the exchange of fresh air in the cabins. Since there is always someone sick on a flight, even the healthiest people tend to develop colds. A friend discovered a personal travel air purifier called Air Supply. She was the only one on her trip to China who didn't develop a respiratory illness. I too have used this tiny device hung around my neck for several transatlantic trips. My eyes were less bloodshot, and so far I haven't caught those dreaded international sniffles.

KIDNEY STONES

Kidney stones are serious. The following traditional remedies should be a supplement to professional medical treatment.

Water Therapy

It is especially important to increase the amount of fluid intake throughout the day to avoid forming kidney stones. For instance, since too much protein increases the calcium in the urine, highly concentrated salts in the urine can crystallize, and they must be flushed out. Therefore, when kidney stones appear, it is urgent to drink 2 to 3 quarts of pure water each day! In this case, constant urination may be the price of freedom.

Drink cranberry juice in addition to drinking water. An experimental study in the journal *Urology* shows that cranberry juice or extract may reduce urinary calcium. One can avoid the sugar in most cranberry juice drinks by taking freeze-dried tablets or capsules. These are obtainable in health food stores.

Rose hip tea appears to be beneficial in reducing calcium oxalate. Drinking raw vegetable juices is also beneficial.

At the turn of the nineteenth-to-the-twentieth century hydrotherapy was used by many outstanding physicians. The early twentieth-century healers George Starr White, M.D. and J. H. Tilden, M.D. praised the following method in the case of an acute attack of kidney stones: Prepare a catnip enema by adding four tablespoons of catnip tea to a quart of warm water. Follow this moderately hot enema with a very hot bath—start at 100°F and increase gradually to 112°F.

Another much touted water healing remedy—this one to induce urination—is a variation on the above. Apply a cold compress to the head and immerse the body in a hot half-bath. Follow the bath with a 1-quart enema, and repeat the enema every 2 hours until urination is possible. While in the hot bath, massage the kidney and bladder area.

To increase urination use any diuretic herbal tea such as parsley, corn silk, goldenrod, juniper berry, rose hip, or dandelion root. To use any of these herbs on a preventive basis, drink a glass of the herb tea each day before lunch. For pain, use a half-cup of any of these natural diuretics every two hours.

For bloody urine, take one small sip an hour of St. John's wort tea.

A macrobiotic remedy is to sip adzuki bean water. Prepare it by adding 1 tablespoon of adzuki beans to 2 quarts of boiling water. Reduce by boiling down to 1 quart. Add a pinch of salt.

General Therapy

A series of acupuncture treatments can often provide relief from various kidney pains.

Magnesium and B_6 are beneficial. Magnesium, especially in magnesium citrate form, helps by making internal calcium oxalate crystals more soluble and consequently easier to excrete. Studies show that a 300 mg dose works well enough; however, experienced medical nutritionists sometimes utilize much larger magnesium citrate doses of up to 1,000 mg. B_6 in daily doses of 50 mg is also useful because it reduces the production of oxalic acid in the body.

Calcium stones can be prevented by reducing the amount of calcium in the bloodstream. Do not, however, go on a low-calcium diet, because your body will react to a permanent lowering of calcium levels by stripping your bones. Increase your intake of fruits and vegetables and high-fiber foods. Maintaining a high-fiber diet that includes whole grains, root vegetables, and beans helps to cut down on calcium excretion. Avoid caffeinated beverages, sugar, salt, and meat products, which promote bursts of calcium excretion that may be a cause of kidney stones. Avoid high-oxalate foods such as spinach, chard, tea, cocoa, and antacids that contain high amounts of calcium, and increase calcium absorption and urinary calcium concentration. Don't drink alcohol or coffee. Avoid all dairy products fortified with vitamin D, which promotes the formation of kidney stones and lowers the magnesium levels in the body.

For uric acid stones eat high-alkaline foods including soy products, fresh fruits and vegetables, avocados, citrus fruits, honey, and corn products. Avoid meats, dairy products, coffee, sweets including soft drinks and chocolate, fast-food condiments such as ketchup, mustard, and relish, all of which are acid-forming foods.

LARYNGITIS

Water Therapy

The double cold compress is a unique comfort to the throat and helps to heal the vocal cords from within. Drink at least 2 quarts of warm water a day to keep the larynx moist. At home keep the air moist with a humidifier.

Aniseeds have a profound effect on laryngitis. The inflamed vocal cords respond to hot anise tea made by bruising some seeds and steeping them in boiling water. Strain out the seeds. The liqueur anisette is also effective. Sip it, or add a teaspoon at a time to a cup of just-boiled water. Chewing aniseeds also helps control the hoarseness.

Continuously drink a hot mash of freshly juiced lemons and lemon rinds plus a substantial amount of honey steeped in just-boiled water. This can be renewed throughout the day. Make sure to thoroughly wash the lemon skins.

For chronic hoarseness use the following long-range water healing techniques to strengthen the body: Tread in cold water up to the ankles several times each day. Apply a cold compress to the chest area several times a week. In addition, sit for a few seconds to several minutes (it will be easier as time goes on) in a cold shallow sit bath several times a week. For chronic conditions, check with a dentist for possible tooth decay or a potential abscess.

General Therapy

Talk as little as possible and don't whisper. Strangely, whispering forces your vocal cords as strongly as does shouting. If you must talk, talk as normally as possible. Carry a pad around to write comments. Suck Slippery Elm lozenges.

The tongue controls laryngitis, and the following pressure exercises are of great help in chronic hoarseness. In private, as frequently as possible, open the mouth wide and thrust out the tongue. Roll it backwards as far as possible, then thrust it out and try to touch the tip of the nose. Cover the upper part of the tongue with a clean handkerchief, squeeze it gently between thumb and forefinger, and pull it around in all directions.

LEG CRAMPS

Water Therapy

Drink at least 2 quarts of water a day. Apply warm compresses to relax cramped muscles.

General Therapy

Prevention: As a preventive measure take supplements of calcium and magnesium, one part calcium to two parts magnesium, as well as a multivitamin that contains 50 mg of B_6 and substantial quantities of vitamins C and E.

During the day take 5 silica 6x cell (tissue) salts under the tongue. Be aware of your electrolyte balance. For potassium, eat bananas, oranges, beans, fresh vegetables, and whole grains. Exercise regularly to improve muscle tone. Wear shoes with good supports during the day. To avoid accumulating fluid in the extremities, experiment with elevating the head or the foot of the bed, or place a small pillow between the knees or on the side. Also keep the bed covers loose. When necessary, wear bed socks to keep the feet warm.

Onset of an Attack: Ingest 5 magnesia phos. 6x cell (tissue) salts under the tongue immediately. The dose can be repeated every 20 minutes, up to 5 doses. Chew some extra tablets to make a paste, and place it directly on the cramp or spasm. When the cramps seem like the creepy, crawly electrical sensations of restless leg syndrome, add 10 to 15 mg of folic acid (some medical nutritionists prescribe doses of up to 60 mg) and small amounts of vitamin B_{12} to the supplement list. For knee cramps, press a point 3 inches above the knee and 3 inches toward the inside of the thigh, maintaining firm pressure for 30 to 90 seconds.

MOUTH SORES

Water Therapy

(Also see "Cold Sores," "Canker Sores," "Dry Mouth") Prepare a mouth rinse by adding 1 teaspoon of salt and 1 teaspoon of hydrogen peroxide to a glass of water.

Rinse the mouth with a glass of water, a few drops of tincture of myrrh, and a pinch of powdered goldenseal. Mouth sores also respond to both of these herbs placed directly on the sore itself.

To avoid an excessively dry mouth, drink copious amounts of water, as much as 10 to 12 glasses a day. To stimulate the flow of saliva, occasionally rinse the mouth with a glass of water diluted with several drops of fresh lemon juice.

General Therapy

Mouth sores in a newborn child may be from a candida infection. Purchase a children's bifidus-acidophilus preparation in the health food store and follow the directions on the package. In addition, massage the child's scalp and torso with flaxseed oil. Keep this oil stored in the refrigerator. Sudden mouth sores in older children may be an indication of an emerging case of chickenpox, measles, scarlet fever, or diphtheria. Check with a physician.

Some painful mouth sores may be caused by highly seasoned foods, alcohol, citrus foods, or tobacco. To avoid an excessively dry mouth, try artificial saliva products such as Salivart, Zero-Lube, Moi-Stir, or Oralbalance. Avoid smoking and drinking alcohol, which can irritate the sensitive membranes in the mouth. Should mouth sores and cracks at the corner of the mouth emerge, the body is showing early signs of a possible B-complex deficiency. Add B-complex supplements to the diet as well as extra B_6 and B_2 (riboflavin), which are specific support remedies for mouth sores and cracks.

NERVOUSNESS

Water Therapy

Long, leisurely, neutral or moderately hot full baths always help to relax the mind and body. Any number of herbs can act as tranquilizers or sedatives, among them hops, passionflower, valerian, catnip, melissa (lemon balm), and oats. Use the herbs singly or in groups. These are so popular in Europe that the Germans produce combinations of the herbs valerian and peppermint, or valerian and melissa, which also help insomnia. Try Zimmermann's famous herbal formula, which combines 30 parts melissa, 20 parts each of angelica and hops, and 10 parts each of rosemary leaf, lavender flower, and yarrow herb. Steep 1 to 2 teaspoons of the combined herbs in 1 cup of boiling water. Steep, strain, and drink 1 to 2 cups before bedtime. Or if the nervousness is due to a stomach upset, take some chamomile or peppermint tea to ease the stomach, or some combination of bitter herbs (like Swedish Bitters) to stimulate the digestive system.

NEURALGIA

FACIAL NEURALGIA

Water Therapy

Spasmodic pain in the face can be alleviated by a hot shower directed at the area of pain. A slightly less effective treatment is a hot water compress applied as hot as can be tolerated to the area of pain.

NEURITIS

Water Therapy

Hot beeswax or hot paraffin treatments are an age-old part of water therapy treatments for localized pain. The paraffin can be purchased by mail (see Resources). Heat about half a cup in a ceramic, glass, or stainless steel pot. A reliable electric "pot" is sold for such purposes. Dip the painful joint or area into the hot paraffin or soak a piece of cotton cloth in the paraffin and apply to the inflamed area. Cover with a slightly larger cotton or light wool cloth to help retain the heat longer. The paraffin makes the area feel very warm and comfortable and relieves the pain. If it feels too hot, peel it off immediately. Otherwise let the heat penetrate, and peel off the wax when it becomes cold.

NOSEBLEED

Water Therapy

Offset dry winter air by adding moisture to the air. Use either fresh pots of water stashed around the room, a cool air mist humidifier, or a hot moist air steam vaporizer.

To stop a nosebleed place an ice pack on the bridge of the nose, and as often as possible apply cold washcloths or ice packs to the back of the neck. As the nosebleed subsides sit with the head leaning back. If no ice or water is available, squeeze the bridge of the nose between the thumb and index finger, or apply strong pressure to the area beneath the nose and above the lips.

If the bleeding won't stop, use witch hazel as a styptic. Dip a rolled piece of absorbent cotton into the liquid extract, squeeze it so it isn't too drippy, and place it in the nose.

General Therapy

During a nosebleed, take 500 mg of vitamin C every 15 minutes for the first hour and 500 mg every half-hour after that until the bleeding stops. To hasten healing apply a thin layer of aloe vera gel or calendula (marigold) ointment inside the nose. If there is a tendency for nosebleeds add substantial amounts of vitamin C and bioflavonoid supplements to the daily diet. Avoid coffee, tea, mint, almonds, cloves, cucumbers, bell peppers, tomatoes, apples, peaches, plums, apricots, cherries, currants, grapes, raisins, and all berries, and be aware that aspirin, blood thinners such as Coumadin or heparin, oral contraceptives and other estrogen supplements, and prolonged use of nosedrops or nasal sprays may contribute to nosebleeds. Frequent nosebleeds may also be an indication of high blood pressure (hypertension).

PAIN

Water Therapy

Ice: Immediately after an injury apply ice to the area of pain or to the nearest artery supplying blood to the area. Ice diminishes pain and prevents blood congealing in the area by reducing blood circulation to the region. Experts have devised the acronym RICE—Rest, Ice, Compression and Elevation—to help us remember what to do in the case of pain, injury, and strains. The Self-Care Catalog carries excellent pliable body-shaped ice wraps for the neck, shoulder, lumbar region, and ankle/elbow. (These wraps can be transformed into heat treatments by heating them in a conventional or microwave oven.)

Heat and Cold: After the initial icing for the first 24 hours, either hot or cold water applications may be used to divert and control the pain: soaks in warm to hot water, application of a hot water bottle, hot water showers directed to the area of the pain, immersing the hands or feet in cold water, ice compresses, a frozen bandage (see page 45), or when indicated, eating ice chips.

Alleviate colicky symptoms with frequent hot cloth compresses placed over the area of the pain.

For minor burns, to deaden the pain and start the healing process, place the burned part of the body in ice water, or apply ice water to the area.

Persistent arthritic pains usually respond to nightly applications of castor oil poultices.

Many pains can be alleviated by applying a neutral clay poultice or a charcoal poultice over the area of the pain.

PERIODONTAL DISEASE

Water Therapy

Spongy, inflamed gums? There is nothing better for a quick recovery than a rinse with tincture of myrrh. Place several drops of the tincture in a quarter-glass of water and thoroughly rinse the problem area. It reduces the inflammation almost immediately, although it may take several days to conquer the entire problem. Tincture of myrrh combined with goldenseal powder makes a dynamic duo. Make into a paste and apply to gums, or add both to water to create a healing mouthwash. Do not swallow this preparation, especially if you are pregnant.

Make up a strong sage leaf tea and store it in a labeled bottle in the refrigerator. Use it as a mouthwash.

Two B vitamins, B$_6$ and folic acid (folate), are especially helpful for periodontal problems, especially those developed during pregnancy. Make up a mouthwash by crushing and dissolving 25 mg of B$_6$ and 2 mg of folic acid supplement into a glass of water. Store in a labeled jar and rinse the mouth frequently. Also include a B-complex vitamin in your daily vitamin regimen.

For centuries, the Japanese have used the humble, pickled umeboshi plum for a wide number of health problems. You can find them at many health food stores. To create a gargle for mouth problems, crush one umeboshi plum and add salt plus 1 cup of boiling water.

General Therapy

In addition to the B-complex, B$_6$, and folic acid mentioned above, include the following crucial supplements in your diet to maintain both general and mouth health: substantial amounts of vitamin C, 400 IU of vitamin E, coenzyme Q10, selenium, and quercetin. Also eat fibrous foods to stimulate the gums. Investigate the following homeopathic cell salt remedies: natrum mur. 6x for gums that are swollen and bleed easily, or if the tongue has ridges and the mouth is dry; and silica 6x for painful swelling and inflammation, boils, or abscesses on the gums or roots of the teeth. For this last problem, do not fail to see a dentist immediately!

PLEURISY

Water Therapy

There are three essential water healing therapies: drinking water, the criss-cross chest compress, and cold water friction massage applied three times a day.

For an Acute Attack: If the right lung is involved, immerse both feet in hot water and apply a hot compress to the right chest. Renew this hot compress as soon as it cools. Repeat up to 5 times. This should relieve the pain. Vigorously rub every other spot on the body except the right lung area with a dry brush, a rough wet washcloth, or a washcloth dipped in apple cider vinegar. Reverse this process for the left lung.

Relief of Pain: Use a cool mist humidifier to ease the coughing and pain while breathing.

Most people find relief from the considerable chest pain of pleurisy with a gentle application of homeopathic arnica ointment, Tiger Balm ointment, camphor oil, or Olbas oil. For thousands of years the Chinese have used ginseng root powder or extract for serious coughs (see "Coughs"). Add some ginseng powder to your favorite herbal tea (such as peppermint) or to hot lemonade. The Chinese also combine ginseng with ginger, licorice root, Chinese angelica (dong quai), and mandarin orange.

Chronic Case: Immerse feet in a hot shallow bath. Apply a hot moist compress to the side of the chest that is involved. Direct a no-force rain spray and alternate hot and cold spray on the chest over the area affected.

Follow the chest spray with alternate hot and cold jet showers directed to the feet and legs. The hot shower should last 4 minutes; the cold shower, 30 seconds. They should be forceful.

Fluids to Flush the System

Drink a substantial amount of water, hot herbal teas, and hot soups to prevent dehydration. Pureed soups not only contain many nutrients, they help boost immune function and encourage profuse perspiration, which helps the body to eliminate toxins. Wear cotton nightclothes to absorb the perspiration, and change the nightclothes as often as possible.

PNEUMONIA

Water Therapy

Before the discovery of antibiotics, many internationally known physicians used water therapy to treat patients who had contracted either bacterial or nonbacterial forms of this acute infection of the lungs. The water therapy did not "attack" the pathogenic aspect of the acute infection, but helped to regenerate the general metabolic system. Hydrotherapists have always looked at the body in a holistic manner and sought to tone the entire body and rebalance its internal energy. This helps nature take over and do most of the healing.

Water treatments for pneumonia, as well as for other acute infections, are directed to stimulating the body's immune system, enlarging the scope of skin elimination, breaking up energy blocks in lungs and elsewhere in the body, and creating tone through circulation.

Because water therapy stimulates the body in an entirely natural way, it undoubtedly hastens the last stage of infection—as in pneumococcal pneumonia when the important "macrophage reaction" takes place. At this time, the mononuclear cells enter the diseased part of the lung, engulf any remaining pneumococci, and phagocytize them. They actually eat up the microorganisms, cellular debris, or foreign particles. It is only when this self-healing process is complete that the X ray will show clear lungs.

A person with pneumonia has an urgent need for absolute rest, fluid therapy, oxygen therapy (sometimes), and body-building water therapy. If desired, after you have learned the exact staph, strep, or bacterial causes, you can use antimicrobial therapy together with the following water treatments. Keep in mind that one strain of pneumonia, *Haemophilus influenzae,* is resistant to the preferred antibiotic therapy.

Water therapy, however, does not replace the need for proper medical care of pneumonia.

Criss-Cross Chest Compress: Tear a large white sheet into strips. Immerse the strips in cold water, wring out, and apply in criss-cross fashion across the chest and back of the patient. Cover the wet compress with dry strips of flannel or wool.

Criss-crossing the cloths allows all portions of the lung to receive the beneficial effect of the cold water. Change the cold strips every 30 minutes, or whenever they become warm and dry. If the patient does not react well, change them more often. The bandages may be left on all night when the patient goes to sleep. To maintain the cold temperature throughout the night, add a layer of oiled silk or plastic over the wet compress (underneath the woolen overwrap).

Cold-Water Friction Massage: Friction-wash each area of the body with cool to cold water. Dry as quickly as possible before going to the next section of the body. Repeat 3 times a day. This sectional washing was developed by Dr. Gustav Nespor, who determined that each series of massages had the same therapeutic action as an 8-minute cold bath. Many persons with pneumonia like this treatment because it overcomes and improves the weakened condition of the body.

If the pulse is weak, apply a cold compress to the heart area every 30 minutes.

Expectoration Aid: Nothing breaks a bad cough faster than an old-fashioned mustard plaster. Prepare it with 1 part of mustard powder to 3 to 4 parts of flour. Add enough tepid water to make it into a paste. Spread the paste onto a thin cotton or flannel "envelope." Shift it around on the chest and back, checking to make sure that the poultice does not blister the skin. For youngsters or adults with sensitive skin, add a light layer of oil or Vaseline before the application.

Still another approach is to use hot compresses applied to the chest and back.

Such compresses act as a counterirritant and break up the congestion by bringing blood to the surface of the skin. This will promote relaxation and increase the discharge of mucus.

Renew the hot compress whenever it cools. Always end this treatment with a brief cold friction massage to restore tonicity of the area. Repeat the entire process every 30 minutes when needed.

These same compresses are also useful in treating bronchitis, asthma of nervous origins, angina pectoris, and other chest conditions.

If mucus is a problem, Dr. Julian Whitaker suggests taking 1 to 2 tablets, three times a day, of Air Power (Enzymatic Therapy), an expectorant that thins the mucus and loosens phlegm and bronchial secretions.

Steam: The patient with bronchial or lobular pneumonia often finds relief when a steam vaporizer is kept going during the day and night.

Mouth and Gums: It is beneficial to gargle and rinse out the mouth and gums with a hot salt solution several times during the day. Another useful gargle is a combination of hot water and glycerin. Use 4 parts hot water to 1 part glycerin.

General Therapy

The patient's room should be very clean, well ventilated, sunny, and kept at a consistent, cool temperature. Since it is important to change positions as often as possible, rig up, borrow, or buy a backrest—the kind with arm rests. The patient will feel better with any of these herbs or oil massages: Tiger Balm, drops of thyme tea or oil, melissa tea or oil, peppermint tea or oil, or wintergreen liniment, added to sesame or olive oil.

POISON IVY, POISON OAK, POISON SUMAC

Water Therapy

If you suspect any contact with any of these three poison plants, do not touch your face or eyes! As soon as possible wash the entire exposed skin area of the hands, feet, and face with hot soapy water—preferably with brown laundry soap. Use gloves, a rag, or a stick to handle shoes, socks, and other clothing. Treat them as if they contain contaminated germs. Clean the shoes several times. Throw away the socks worn at the time of contact.

When the itching starts, apply either witch hazel or plain cold compresses. Throw away the contaminated cloths. Run very hot water over the sores. This usually relieves the itchiness for about a half-hour at a time.

Oatmeal and/or apple cider vinegar greatly relieves the itchiness. Alternate long, leisurely hot baths in either finely ground oatmeal particles or

Aveeno, colloidal oatmeal purchased at the drugstore, or baths containing 1 to 2 cups of apple cider vinegar.

General Therapy

If you have touched poison ivy, look for a nearby stand of yellow-flowered jewelweed (*Impatiens biflora*). In the spring, the juice from the stems of the jewelweed plant can be used to wash off poison ivy toxins, usually reducing the virulence of an attack. A remarkable antidote to poison ivy, the homeopathic rhus tox. remedy usually works immediately. Follow the specific directions for adult and child doses. If it isn't available, use any of the following for the itching: the gel from a living aloe vera plant, calendula (marigold) homeopathic ointment, or calamine lotion, a substance that also dries the sores. Also, to dispel the repulsive feeling of contamination, place a few drops of Crabapple, one of the 38 Bach Flower Remedies, under the tongue.

PSORIASIS

Psoriasis remains an unpredictable and perplexing disease. There are a variety of approaches to contain the condition.

Water Therapy

Proper digestion and elimination are essential in controlling psoriasis. Each morning, to control possible constipation, drink 2 glasses of room-temperature cold water. (Also read "Constipation.")

In Europe, "wet on wet" is the traditional approach to weeping and inflamed skin diseases. Early stages of both psoriasis and eczema respond quickly to rapid replacement compresses consisting of one of two herbs: the astringent oak bark (*Quercus* sp.) or mucilaginous (soft and gummy) plants such as high mallow (*Malva sylvestris*) or dwarf mallow (*Malva neglecta*), and later in the dry stage, antiseptic and anti-inflammatory chamomile, a common herbal table tea.

At the early wet stage, each day prepare a fresh batch of a solution of oak bark by simmering 1 to 2 tablespoons of chopped oak bark in 1 quart of water for 20 minutes. Strain out the bark, cool the liquid, plunge in the compress material, wring it out, and apply it to the weeping sores. The oak bark has also proved effective for eczema and leg ulcers arising from this condition. Make mallow solutions in the same way as the oak bark.

In the dry stage use either chamomile ointment such as CamoCare (Abit) or Simicort (Enzymatic Therapy), which contains licorice and the skin-healing substance allantoin, or chamomile tea combined with zinc oxide ointment. Zinc oxide ointment may also be combined with either avocado oil or 2 to 5 percent St. John's wort oil. After the dry stage, many German physicians also prescribe a low percent of juniper tar delivered to the sores with zinc oxide ointment. Tar applications, which also include tar from birch, beech, or pine trees, must be carefully monitored for possible skin irritations.

Each year, thousands of psoriasis victims help to control future attacks with a week or two at an Israeli Dead Sea resort. Soaking in the heavily salted Dead Sea seems to give victims a six-month period of freedom from attacks. If this is not possible and the above herbal remedies are not used, try to daub the sores with compresses saturated with Dead Sea salts, mineral salts, or common salt (keep applications hot by covering with a dry cloth). Or try for the same effect as continuous soaking in the Dead Sea with a series of brief hot baths (temperature 100°F to 102°F) that are saturated with large quantities of Dead Sea salts, mineral salts, or table salt. End each brief bath with a fleeting cold shower. It also helps to bathe in the ocean and to take moderate advantage of sunny weather to dry up the sores.

Some, but not all, psoriasis patients respond to brief baths that contain 1 cup of either apple cider vinegar or ascorbic acid crystals.

General Therapy

Some clinical studies suggest that psoriasis may be due to a marginal liver malfunction. To protect liver function, it is essential to avoid drinking alcohol. One liver-helping plant is milk thistle (*Silybum marianum*), the first choice of modern herbalists and physicians who use plants for psoriasis therapy. Milk thistle is now produced in a standardized capsule. The dose can range from 70 mg up and is usually taken 3 times a day. Some patients also do well on a daily regimen of lecithin granules (avoid the capsules, because they are not well absorbed). Other causes of flareups may be yeast infections, which occur after eating sugar products. Many patients appear to need metabolic boosting from essential fatty acids. These can be obtained by eating sardines, salmon, herring, mackerel, and nuts, especially walnuts.

Some alternative practitioners have success prescribing capsules or 3 table-spoons of flaxseed each day. Flaxseed intake should be balanced with vitamin E intake to offset the formation of free radicals.

RINGWORM

Water Therapy

During ringworm outbreaks take particular care to wash and disinfect the hands throughout the day. Also wash children's clothes every day.

Each day during an outbreak liberally apply tea tree oil diluted with distilled water to the ring-shaped rash until the rash disappears. To use this impressive disinfectant and antifungal Australian herb, combine 8 drops of the oil and 2 glasses of water (preferably distilled water). Apply with a disposable cotton swab or cloth.

If tea tree oil is not available, apply fresh-squeezed lemon juice to the area of the skin affected with ringworm. The lemon may be lightly diluted with water.

General Therapy

Ringworm is contagious! Do not allow children to share combs, hairbrushes, hats, scarves, pillowcases, or bed sheets. Avoid touching dogs, cats, or other pets with telltale ring-shaped hairless patches. To boost the body's healing ability and help overcome stress, add echinacea on a 10-day on, 10-day off schedule, and add high amounts of vitamin C supplements and foods to the diet. A Western folk medicine cure for ringworm: Light a match and while it is still burning, place it in a saucer. Scrape the yellow film deposit of the burned match onto a cotton swab and apply it directly to the ringworm patch. Repeat this burned match and swabbing procedure several times each day.

ROSACEA

Water Therapy

Two times a day apply very hot moist compresses directly to the lesions, touching each lesion 5 or 6 times. However, avoid putting hot towels directly on the face.

Drink plenty of water throughout the day.

Take a leisurely neutral-hot bath (about 102°F). Add 1 ounce of potassium sulphate (homeopathic sulphur) to the bathwater. Gently pat the skin dry with a soft cotton or flannel cloth.

General Therapy

Do not engage in too many activities or exercises that will bring blood to the surface of the skin, drink alcohol or coffee, or eat steamy or excessively hot or spicy foods that flush the face. Also avoid hot tubs, steam rooms, saunas, steam facials, and hot towels to the face. Avoid sunlight. If you are on antibiotic therapy, counteract its automatic depletion of intestinal flora by consuming a high-potency lactobacillus acidophilus capsule or yogurt. Avoid medicated acne products, which may irritate the rosacea, as well as cortisone creams or ointments, or cosmetics, moisturizers, sunscreens or aftershave products that contain alcohol. If you intend to get pregnant, stop using the acne medicine Accutane, and if you are pregnant, after the second month avoid using the antibiotic tetracycline, since this may damage the bones and teeth of the fetus.

Clinical studies show that B-complex vitamins, especially riboflavin and B_6, are useful therapies. One study showed that pancreatic enzymes taken internally both diminish the lesions and reduce digestive problems. Some digestive problems may occur because of a reduced output of hydrochloric acid, a situation that often occurs with rosacea patients. As for migraine headaches, which sometimes occur, investigators surmise they may be due to a food sensitivity problem. To test this, eliminate one food at a time for one to two weeks, then challenge the body with that food to see if there is an allergic reaction, unusual behavior, or uncommon fatigue. Holistic experts also suggest eliminating animal product foods and concentrating on a vegetarian diet, or combining a vegetarian with a fruit diet.

SCARS

Water Therapy

Ancient Chinese medical practitioners washed scars with cherry seeds boiled in water. To boost healing from within the body, drink honey-laced lemonade, eat pineapple, and drink pineapple juice as well as bromelain, the pineapple enzyme available as a supplement. Also drink carrot and celery as well as other vegetable juices.

General Therapy

Take vitamin E internally. Apply pricked-open capsules of vitamin E (consisting of pure alpha d' (not dl) tocopherol, day after day to the scar until it diminishes. Vitamin E is the best external ointment, but homeopathic calendula ointment made from marigolds and aloe vera gel slit from the leaf of the plant also help to heal scars and may be applied on a regular basis.

SCIATICA

Water Therapy

As soon as possible after an initial attack, apply a cold pack to the area of the buttocks most in pain. After 15 minutes apply another cold pack to the area of the leg most in pain.

If you are prone to sciatic attacks, always have some "frozen bandages" ready in the freezer. To prepare, dip three to four soft, old washcloths in cold water. Wring out. Flatten out and fold in two. Place in a plastic bag a little larger than the folded washcloth. Stack a series of these wet, folded cloths on a flat cardboard in the freezer. When a sciatic spasm occurs, lie directly on the frozen washcloth. Before long the body will send heat to the area, and the frozen washcloth will become limp and hot. Replace it immediately with a fresh, frozen one. It normally takes two such applications to alleviate a spasm, but be prepared for a longer treatment.

If the situation becomes a chronic problem, use alternate (long) hot and (brief) cold applications to the area of the pain, always ending with the cold spurt. Such applications can include hot and cold shower sprays, hot and cold compresses, hot whirlpool plunges, or brief cold pool dips.

General Therapy

Several slow stretches help to lessen the pain. One that seems difficult, but is amazingly effective in unkinking the spasm, is the slow leg lift and equally slow stretch across the body: Lie on your back. Lift the leg on the same side as the sciatic attack and slowly stretch it upward and across the body toward the opposite shoulder.

Strengthen the abdominal muscles with partial shoulder situps. Lie on the floor with knees bent and hands behind your head. Keep the back pressed against the floor and lift the shoulders up a dozen times. Repeat as often as possible during the day. Another abdominal strengthener is to stand with hands on hips, bending the upper body in a fluid circle forward, right, backwards, and left. Reverse the circle. Repeat 5 to 10 times, several times a week.

To strengthen and soothe the back, lie on the floor, lift the legs and rest the knees on a couch or chair. This is a very restful pose and can be done even when watching TV.

SHINGLES

Shingles is an acute infection of the central nervous system that is characterized by eruptions and neuralgic pains. It is caused by a virus, and though it may happen to anyone, it is most common in people over fifty. One attack usually confers immunity.

Water Therapy

To provide temporary relief from the agonizing pain of shingles, have someone gently massage your back and spinal column until you discover an extremely sensitive or painful area. Place two towels on the bed, and lie with the painful area directly on an ice cube or cold pack.

Take frequent, long, leisurely, warm to hot baths. To ease the misery of the blisters, add 1 cup of soothing colloidal oatmeal (Aveeno) to the bathwater. A cup of apple cider vinegar may be added to any nonoatmeal bath.

Slit open a leaf of an aloe vera plant and apply the gel to the blisters.

An over-the counter cayenne pepper or capsaicin ointment may be applied directly to the blisters to ease the nerve pain. This type of preparation takes about 10 days to become entirely effective, but it has a remarkably positive effect. It comes in two strengths. Purchase the stronger one.

General Therapy

In general, avoid extreme stress. The herpes zoster virus (childhood chickenpox) hides in the nerve ganglia and reemerges as blister-type eruptions when a patient is overstressed or overtired. Because the pain is on the nerve pathway it can be agonizing. If you suspect an attack (shingles occur on only one side of the body, and the pustules can be confused with an outbreak of poison ivy), immediately check in with your physician for a proper diagnosis, and request (not every doctor prescribes it automatically) the antiviral acyclovir, i.e., Zovirax, to inactivate the virus, quicken the healing, and lessen the possibility of postherpetic neuralgia, a condition that can plague one for years.

Boost your all immune functions with vitamin C supplements spaced out during the day, echinacea tablets or liquid extracts, and high doses of B-complex supplements that contain vital B_{12}, a singular antishingles aid. Some doctors will give patients shots of B_{12} during this period. Otherwise, supplementation with 500 mg of B_{12} has proved helpful. To further lessen the possibility of postherpetic neuralgia take daily supplements of vitamin E.

During periods of stress calm down with conscious deep breathing alternated with yoga alternate nostril breathing. With the thumb cover the right nostril and to the count of 4 breathe in through the left nostril. Breathe out through the right nostril to the count of 4. Repeat several times. This immediately reduces stress and tension and brings on a benign feeling.

The pain and misery of a shingles attack are legendary. Practice positive affirmations by telling yourself again and again, "I feel good," "I don't have anything to worry about," "This too will pass, and everything will turn out fine."

SINUS INFECTION

Water Therapy

Moisture is an essential and effective way to expel the thick, uncomfortable mucus in the sinus that results from an infection in the sinus area.

To alleviate pain apply a series of hot compresses over your closed eyes and to the entire nasal and sinus area, the hotter the better. To deepen the effectiveness of these applications add drops of rosemary tea or oil, peppermint tea or oil, or the essential oil of oregano (*Origanum vulgare*) to the compress water. A colleague, Bernard Asbell, swears by still another hot, moist application. He uses a hot water bottle on the painful area.

To improve drainage and lessen the pain of a sinus attack breathe in steam—run a shower in a closed bathroom, or improvise a steam tent with a pot of boiling water placed on a safe, nonwobbly table. Create a tent with a large towel. Close your eyes and place your head under the towel, and breathe in the cleansing steam. It is beneficial to add the following herbs to any steaming water: pine, eucalyptus, rosemary, chamomile, peppermint, or wild oregano. Wild oregano also comes in capsule form, and many patients report it is effective in reducing a sinus infection.

One of the best preventive approaches is inhaling a daily saline (salt water) solution. Do this often, says the holistic physician Dr. Robert S. Ivker, former president of the American Holistic Medical Association and author of the excellent book, *Sinus Survival*. It can control the tendency to get sinus infections. If fighting an infection, repeat this sniffing up to 4 times a day. Use an eyedropper for small children. Indian Ayurvedic practitioners often add a pinch of the herb turmeric, a powerful anti-inflammatory, to the saline solution. American naturopaths add a few grains of powdered goldenseal to this nasal douche, and also advise using either a freeze-dried capsule, tincture, powder, or extract of the herb internally to counter bacterial infections. Do not use goldenseal if you are pregnant or planning a pregnancy since it may cause uterine contractions.

Moisture restores normal cilia function in the nose and relieves nasal and head congestion, headaches, sinus pain, and sore throats. Mix $\frac{1}{3}$ of a teaspoon of noniodized table salt with a touch of baking soda to 1 cup of lukewarm bottled water. The combination makes the solution close to the healthy body's salinity and pH, which makes the procedure more comfortable than if you were to use plain water. Use half a cup of the solution for each nostril. With the head in an upright position, pinch one nostril while pouring the solution into the other nostril. For this procedure, you can use a large, all-rubber ear syringe; the palm of your hand (simply sniff the solution up your nose); a Neti pot, which is a porcelain pot with a narrow spout (see Resources) that comes from Ayurvedic medicine; or an eyedropper for a small child. Repeat the procedure 1 to 4 times a day, depending on the severity of the condition. Nasal irrigation is also a good remedy for chronic sinusitis sufferers, who are often vexed with dry, crusted nasal membranes that make them more susceptible to nosebleeds.

To soothe the system, increase healing, and drain the mucus during an attack, drink lots of thin, clear, hot liquids such as hot lemonade with honey and substantial quantities of clear chicken soup.

For sinus problems, Dr. Aaron M. Flickstein of Minneapolis, Minnesota prescribes a mycelized version of vitamin A because of vitamin A's importance in skin cell regeneration. Flickstein tells his patients to combine the liquid vitamin with water on a $\frac{1}{10}$ to a $\frac{1}{3}$ ratio of vitamin A to water in an empty spray bottle, a dropper bottle, or a Neti pot. During an acute attack, spray or insert the solution into the nostrils four times a day. Flickstein reports, "So far every patient with sinus infection or inflammation has obtained dramatic and rapid healing using this approach."

The following compress is an old Italian remedy for a sinus attack. Chop one medium onion and place it on a piece of gauze. Place the gauze on a longer and wider cotton cloth and wrap it around the throat. Close with a safety pin. Leave the compress on all night to draw out the infection from the nasal passages.

General Therapy

During an attack do not blow each nostril separately, because this is likely to send the mucus back into the sinus cavities. Instead gently blow the nose with both nostrils simultaneously.

Acute sinusitis, which lasts a month or less, is typically caused by a bacteria. Chronic sinusitis, an inflammation of the membranes of the nose and sinus cavities that lasts three months or longer, affects about 37 million Americans each year. Until recently, it was considered a bacterial infection. However, according to recent research at the Mayo Clinic, 90 percent of cases are probably caused by an immune-system response to a common fungus. If you are prone to sinus attacks, bolster your immune system with a 10-day on, 10-day off regimen of echinacea.

If attacks come regularly, investigate the possibility of sensitivity to one or more foods. If eliminating mucus-producing dairy products doesn't work, check other food sensitivities one by one. Since marginal nutritional deficiencies can also contribute to serial sinus attacks, Dr. Julian Whitaker recommends taking 1,000 mg of vitamin C or "as much as your bowel will tolerate every waking hour" (diarrhea occurs at the point the body has enough, or more than enough vitamin C). Suck on one or two (no more) zinc lozenges and one dose of beta-carotene each day, and eat vitamin A–rich yellow and orange foods and vitamin C foods during an attack. Since garlic is a powerful antibactericide, add fresh, mashed garlic to salads and other foods. Swallow one or two garlic capsules each day.

To shift the mucus out of the throat and away from the ears, vigorously massage the foot area under the toes. Start each massage under the little toe and work toward the large toe.

Two homeopathic remedies used throughout Europe are hepar sulph. 3x and cinnabaris 3x, both of which the naturopath Dr. Amos Vogel believes eliminate the pus and heal the affected part. Using them, says Vogel, "makes syringing the nasal passages superfluous."

SORE THROAT

A sore throat (also see "Tonsillitis"), which is a symptom, not a disease, is usually advance notice of an upcoming cold or a threatening viral or bacterial infection. Attacking the symptom of a sore throat is smart medicine and helps to avert a more dangerous health problem. Water healing solutions vary from gargles to compress wraps.

Water Therapy

Moderate Sore Throat: Salt-water gargling is a first line of defense. In addition you can also gargle with apple cider vinegar diluted with water, or sherry wine to which cinnamon and/or caraway seeds have been added.

Nothing suits an early sore throat better than a double throat compress, which incorporates a wet, cold compress fastened around the neck and a second wool compress over it to trap the cold. The body reacts to the cold by sending blood rushing to the area. Because the cold is "trapped" by the wool, the compress heats up from within, which not only feels comforting, but is the beginning of a natural healing process. Renew this compress as soon as it gets warm.

Still another effective double throat compress combines two layers of brown paper (a brown bag or wrapping paper), each soaked in a combination of 1 part wintergreen oil to 6 parts apple cider vinegar (optional: add a pinch of cayenne pepper). Shake off excess fluid and wind the paper as a bandage around the neck. Cover with a long cotton cloth. Fasten with a safety pin. Wear all night long.

For centuries Native Americans and, later, early pioneers in the West used hot sage gargles to offset throat soreness. Sage (*Salvia officinalis*) is extremely antiseptic and can soothe a tough sore throat within minutes. This sage tea can also be used as a soothing drink and as a mouthwash.

Any respiratory infection calls for a ginger treat. Steep shaved ginger-root in hot water, cooled peppermint tea, or carbonated seltzer and use as a gargle. Ginger can also be added to cereals, grains, vegetables, soup, or fruit. Another way to use ginger is to suck on crystallized ginger candy. The sugar can be soaked off—the ginger is still biting and delicious.

Citrus fruits, which are high in vitamin C, help to fight infection. An old favorite for both laryngitis and sore throat is a combination of soothing hot lemonade and honey, drunk throughout the day. Scrub the outside rinds of 4 lemons. Cut them open and squeeze the juice into 1 quart of water. Add the clean rinds. Bring to a light boil. Pour into a large pitcher. Dissolve several tablespoons of honey into the hot lemonade. Refresh throughout the day with extra hot water, some honey, and one or two lemons.

The white pith of the grapefruit is high in needed bioflavonoids. Add some pith to your grapefruit juice.

Vitamin A vegetables are also anti-infection aids. One glass of freshly extracted carrot juice contains about 17,000 IU of vitamin A. Alternate the carrot juice with occasional drinks of juiced mixed green vegetables combined with carrot.

The ancient Egyptians taught us the value of figs as medicine. Boil 2 ounces of figs in 2 cups of boiling water. Cool, strain out the figs, and gargle with the water. The figs may be eaten separately and will help to overcome constipation.

Severe Sore Throat: Take away the congestion by a combination of reflex and depletion techniques.

1. Soak cloths in apple cider vinegar and wind around the feet. Soon the feet will feel very hot as the bandage draws blood from the throat to the feet.

2. Soak a cloth that has been folded several times in apple cider vinegar, wring it out thoroughly, and apply to the abdomen. Renew as soon as it gets warm. This is important, because when the compress gets hot, the blood will again flow in the direction of the throat and the inflammation will return. This compress reinforces the action of drawing the blood away from the throat and thus decreases the inflammation, and it also increases the extraction of toxic material.
3. Soak a cloth in cold water, wring it out thoroughly, and apply it to the neck. Renew it as soon as it becomes warm. Be sure to keep the water from dripping on the chest. Also, keep the rest of the body covered and protected.

General Therapy

Two different lozenges are very effective for sore throats. Slippery Elm lozenges manufactured by Thayer are most soothing. Also try zinc lozenges or zinc combined with vitamin C. Two should be enough. Add vitamin C tablets throughout the day.

A reflexology point for sore throat is the fleshy part of the big toe. Press deeply and massage the toe with the hands or the eraser end of a pencil.

STIFF NECK

Water Therapy

A double throat compress of brown paper soaked in wintergreen oil and apple cider vinegar is a powerful remedy for a stiff neck. For instructions on how to prepare the compress, see the section on sore throats.

TAPEWORM

Water Therapy

The following simple folk remedy for expelling tapeworms from the intestines has proved successful for many people: At night, before going to bed, take an herbal laxative such as Inner Clean or Swiss Kriss. Skip breakfast in the morning. Upon arising, crush pumpkin seeds into a powder using a nut grinder or a food processor. Place the powder in 4 quarts of water and bring to a light boil for half an hour. Drink 6 ounces of the mixture every half-hour. This should expel the tapeworm in several hours.

TEMPOROMANDIBULAR DISORDERS

TMD, or temporomandibular disorders, cause minor to severe pain in the temporomandibular joint (TMJ), which is the hinge joint on each side of the head where the lower jawbone connects with the temporal bone of the skull. There are a variety of causes for the condition, ranging from arthritis to tension, which makes the jaw clench and overuse the supporting TMJ muscles.

Water Therapy

Experiment with cold or hot compresses to the jaw to see which works best for you, or apply ice and then moist heat to the jaw.

General Therapy

Gentle exercises, such as rolling the head in a circle, are good for relaxing the neck. It is important to rest your jaw as much as possible and avoid chewing gum or chewy foods.

TONSILLITIS

Inflamed tonsils feel like a severe sore throat and may produce a high fever and a health crisis.

Water Therapy

There are several approaches that help tonsillitis. The most important of the water therapy strategies involves several simultaneous water actions. One produces perspiration and thereby helps eliminate toxins; the other provides a positive tonic affect.

Heat to the Legs: to prevent feeling chilly, cover the upper torso with some towels. Get into bed under the covers to perspire and apply hot, moist compresses to the legs. (Or take a brief hot leg bath, and then rush under the bed covers.)

Heat to the Throat: While in bed, apply a hot, moist compress to the throat.

To offset the natural weakness brought on by the hot compresses, use ice packs simultaneously applied to the top and sides of the head, and an ice pack to the heart.

Stay in bed about an hour to perspire. Have a helper occasionally exchange the hot leg compresses to induce additional perspiration. After an hour, take a tepid shower or bath. Avoid chilling the body.

Tonic Measures: Vigorously rub the entire body, section by section (keep unexposed areas covered) with a cold, wet, rough washcloth. If possible add a half to a full cup of apple cider vinegar to the cold water.

Heating the Glands of the Neck: Make up a triangle of clean cotton cloth. Dip into apple cider vinegar and apply to the neck and chest. Cover completely with a larger, soft wool blanket. Dip another, longer strip of cotton into apple cider vinegar, wring it out, wind from the chin past the area of the ears, and fasten on the top of the head. Cover the wet compress with a long, dry, soft wool scarf. These two double compresses, one wet, the other dry, will marshall heat resources from within the body and help to break the congestion in the tonsils and throat.

Several times a day, 15 minutes at a time, apply an ice bag to the carotid arteries on the neck (the arteries from the middle of the neck upwards to the side of the chin).

Steam: Use medicated steam in a vaporizer to ease the pain of the throat. Add either eucalyptus oil, pine oil, or drops of tincture of benzoin to the vaporizer well.

Throat Compresses: Combine 3 ounces of deodorized castor oil and 2 drops of camphorated oil. Dip a long folded cotton or flannel cloth into the oils. Wring it out. Apply as a bandage to the throat. Fasten with a safety pin. Apply and fasten a larger but light cotton cloth over the first one. Go to sleep with this compress. This compress will also work for swollen glands, a stiff neck, and the mumps.

Blackberry tea plus apple cider vinegar, or plain blackberry vinegar is an excellent poultice for a severe sore throat. Dip a long folded cotton cloth in the tea or vinegar, wring it out, and apply as a bandage to the throat. Cover completely with a wool scarf.

See "Sore Throat" section for brown paper and wintergreen–apple cider vinegar throat compress.

Gargles: Many common household substances may be used as gargles. Cayenne pepper powder is used throughout the world against a malignant sore throat. Add a pinch of cayenne to water, pineapple juice, or lemonade and gargle. Common table salt can be dissolved into a gargle that can be used throughout the day. Blackberry juice or jelly can be added to water or peppermint tea for a gargle (and a drink) throughout the day. Honey and apple cider vinegar and water may be combined for an excellent gargle. Pineapple juice may be used as a gargle to reduce inflammation.

Master herbalists favor the astringent bayberry bark gargle to clear all morbid matter from the throat. Simmer 1 teaspoon of bayberry bark in 1 pint of boiling water for half an hour. Strain out the bark and gurgle the water in the throat.

General Therapy

At the turn of the twentieth century ear, nose, and throat physician Dr. William Fitzgerald developed a touch therapy he named Zone Therapy. He showed his patients two control points to press to alleviate pain and discomfort: the sides of the tongue, and the joints of the second, third, and fourth fingers of each hand.

ULCERS

Water Therapy

Ulcers are painful sores in the stomach lining or duodenum. Ulcers are caused by a host of factors, such as smoking, alcohol, and stress.

Drinking plenty of water is beneficial to the entire digestive system and is particularly helpful for ulcers. A doctor treating prisoners in jail without the benefit of medication found that the patients' ulcer pains lessened within 3 to 8 minutes of their drinking a glass of water.

Drinking about a quart of cabbage juice daily allows ulcers to heal rapidly.

If bleeding is present, apply ice bags over the stomach and chew tiny bits of cracked ice.

URINATION

Water Therapy

An improvised upward-directed herbal steam bath is an effective treatment to stimulate the flow of urine. To a 3- to 4-quart pot, add a handful of chamomile, oatstraw, or horsetail dried herb and boiling water. Place the steaming pot in the toilet and, being careful not to have the steam too hot so that it will burn, sit above the rising steam. Retain the steam flow by wrapping a large towel or blanket around the body. Or place a stool in the bathtub and put the steaming pot under the stool. Cover the body with a blanket and allow the steam to envelope the lower extremities.

Kneipp and the other early masters of hydrotherapy also had patients sit in warm oatstraw or horsetail baths, and also advised drinking either oatstraw, horsetail, juniper berry, or rose hip tea.

part 4
Water Healing for Men, Women, and Children

WATER HEALING FOR MEN

FERTILITY AND HOT BATHS

Excess heat impairs fertility because of its effect on the testicles and their sperm-producing powers. Some families have trouble conceiving because the men take hot baths for backaches or relaxation, or they work in hot bakeries or near industrial ovens. While trying to conceive, men should avoid very hot baths, hot whirlpools and saunas, even wearing a rubber sweatsuit. For men whose work is continuously hot and hazardous, urologist Dr. Adrian Zorgniotti of New York University School of Medicine has devised a scrotal cooler, which is worn like a jockstrap.

PROSTATE PROBLEMS

Prostatitis is a frustrating and painful condition in which the prostate becomes enlarged, making urination difficult.

PREVENTION

Water Therapy

Drink substantial amounts of pure water. Avoid rich foods that are high in fats and drinking alcohol. Control constipation and/or indigestion.

General Therapy

Although the causative factors of prostate problems are elusive, nutritional and mineral deficiencies contribute to the problem. The prostate gland contains a substantial quantity of zinc. Sometimes a marginal deficiency in zinc contributes to either enlargement (BPH: benign prostatic hyperplasia) and/or an inflamed or infected prostate (prostatitis). Foods rich in zinc are eggs, oysters, herring, brewer's yeast, squash, sesame seeds, tahini (made from sesame seeds), almonds, and molasses. To make sure of an adequate supply of zinc, eat one-quarter to a half-cup of pumpkin seeds each day. Twice each day take saw palmetto berry extract, an herb that has been used for several centuries to alleviate prostate difficulties. Presently, its use is considered so helpful that saw palmetto has strayed into mainstream medicine. Because of its initial clinical use in Germany, the berries are now available in purified form. The usual prescription is 160 mg, 2 times a day.

PAIN

Water Therapy

This is one of the few cases in which either hot or cold applications can work. Initially, use only one or the other.

ACUTE STAGE

Hot Applications

Sit in a brief hot shallow sitz bath. Add strong chamomile tea to this bath.

Immerse the feet in a hot, shallow footbath.

For acute cases, early American masters of water therapy healing usually advised taking a series of hot enemas.

Cold Applications

Apply an ice bag continuously to the area. Take a series of cold-water enemas.

CHRONIC PROBLEM

Water Therapy

After the acute stage of inflammation ends, apply either alternate brief hot and cold compresses or alternate hot and brief cold showers, particularly to the area between the anus and the scrotum, an area exquisitely sensitive to the ministrations of water therapy. Reports indicate that chronic cases that have resisted all sorts of medications respond readily to water therapy treatments.

Another excellent treatment is the graduated 6-minute cold shallow bath, which should start at a temperature of 98°F and gradually decrease in temperature to 75°F. Whenever possible add sea minerals such as salt and kelp to the water. Always end cold sit baths with an alternate hot and cold perineal (area between the anus and the scrotum) spray.

Make a healing tea of corn silk, 1 cup of boiling water to 1 tablespoon of the fresh silk, or a half-tablespoon of the dried silk. Steep for 20 minutes, then strain out the silk. The fresh or dried corn silk may also be applied directly to the genital area to sooth and reduce pain.

Some naturopathic European physicians have had success combining herbal steam baths with the Swiss herbal preparation Prostasan. Clinical studies show that after the series of baths, the prostate usually returns to its normal size. However, there are frequent relapses unless the treatment is continued, usually using about one-third of the original early dosage.

General Therapy

For chronic prostatitis, the eminent holistic physician Dr. Julian Whitaker prescribes 150 mg of zinc for a month, and 45 mg thereafter. Other foods and supplements useful for prostatitis are echinacea to improve immune function, essential fatty acids, vitamin E, magnesium, B complex, vitamin B₆, carrot juice, lemon juice, and water. Avoid dairy products, caffeine, alcohol, high-fat foods, and citrus fruits.

An alternative route away from antibiotics, one that many holistic physicians have used successfully, is to use a special preparation of goldenseal, an herb that contains berberine, a powerful compound that is strongly antibacterial and antifungal. The downside of goldenseal is that its action is much slower than an antibiotic, but there are no presently known side effects to its use. It has the added advantage of stimulating the immune system. Dr. Whitaker prescribes Hydrastine (Enzymatic Therapy), which contains goldenseal and an enzymatic buffer, bromelain, in doses of 2 to 4 capsules, 3 times a day between meals along with a large glass of water. The reason antibiotics are sometimes needed is that the infection and inflammation of prostatitis may be caused by chlamydia. Should an antibiotic be prescribed, also use 400 mg of bromelain enzyme 3 times a day on an empty stomach. This reinforces the effectiveness of the antibiotic. To counter the destruction of good bacteria in the digestive tract, also take capsules or a "living" yogurt containing lactobacillus acidophilus.

SEXUAL LASSITUDE

In a world with Viagra and other quick fixes, some may wonder why anyone would bother with any other resources. Undoubtedly, men who experience a diminishing of sexual energy or impotence should have a physician evaluate them for potential vascular, neurological, and hormonal malfunctions as well as to discuss life stressors, performance anxiety, and possible relationship or marital discord. An effective physician can help you overcome all or most of these problems, and redirect a change of lifestyle as well as the possible replacement of missing nutrients.

Water Therapy

The great hydrotherapists of the past recommended cold-water treatments to overcome sexual lassitude. The following stimulating water therapies are most beneficial: a quick (brief) immersion in a full cold bath; vigorous streams of cold water directed to the spine; or a few seconds' dip in a shallow (6 to 8 inches) sitz bath with the feet in a pan of hot water. This last immersion is frequently done at a spa, which usually has a special bathtub, and a helper massages the hips and back of the person in the tub.

Here's how to prepare the body for the necessary cold treatments: Run some cold water in the bathtub and immerse a big toe a few seconds at time, gradually increasing the time to several minutes. Another approach includes ending every shower with a brief burst of cold water. The whole approach is to be continued until the fear of extreme cold evaporates and contact with the cold becomes an easy and pleasurable event.

The great Finnish naturopath Paavo Airola suggested this blended drink rich in B-complex foods to help overcome sexual exhaustion. Certain foods are necessary for sexual ardor, and this drink includes them all—folic acid– and B$_6$-rich foods as well as zinc and magnesium foods.

In a blender grind 2 ice cubes, 2 tablespoons of pumpkin seeds, 2 tablespoons of lecithin granules, and 1 tablespoon of sesame seeds. To this add 1½ glasses of whole milk (Airola likes goat milk in particular), 2 tablespoons of skim milk powder, 1 tablespoon of honey, two (organic) egg yolks (the Country Hen brand from Maine is high in omega-3 nutrients) and 1 tablespoon of wheat germ oil. Add another ice cube if you wish. Blend the mixture together. The ice creates a pleasant foam and the drink can be eaten with a spoon.

General Therapy

In addition to the B-complex-rich foods, drink freshly made vegetable juices with an emphasis on carrot combinations such as carrot and celery, carrot and spinach, and carrot blended with wheat germ and the seaweed dulse or kelp. Ginseng powder and extract is used throughout Asia to overcome sexual weariness. Another Asian remedy to overcome sexual depletion is to eat the meat of 6 walnuts each day for 2 months. In Louisiana, men restore themselves with a three-week diet that includes eating a handful of fresh-cooked shrimp and a small shot of brandy each day. Other foods of the sea are excellent for changing sexual fatigue to sexual energy: eat crab, lobster, shrimp, oysters, mussels, ocean fish, and seaweed such as kelp and dulse. In ancient Europe, oatmeal was a favored diet to repair sexual apathy.

SPERMATORRHEA (INVOLUNTARY DISCHARGE OF SEMEN)

Water Therapy

To check spermatorrhea (the involuntary loss of semen), direct a 2-minute cold jet spray to the soles of the feet. Do this daily.

Rest the base of the skull on a bag of crushed ice and rock salt for a prolonged time. This inhibits activity in the genital area.

Note: Short applications of ice will, by reflex action, stimulate the sexual organs. Also, consider using a genital compress.

TESTICULAR INFLAMMATION (ORCHITIS)

Orchitis is an inflammation of the testicles that is generally caused by germs carried in the bloodstream. The inflammation should not be neglected, because it can eventually cause infertility.

Water Therapy

Shore up the immune system by taking 10 to 20 drops of echinacea tincture, tablets, or spray every hour. Go on a 10-day on, 10-day off schedule.

Avoid constipation by drinking 2 glasses of room-temperature water on arising each morning and drinking massive amounts of water throughout the day.

At night before going to bed, combine a handful of healing neutral clay, several tablespoons of high-silica horsetail tea, plus a tablespoon of St. John's wort oil to keep the clay moist. Apply this wet mudpack to the inflamed area. When the clay or soil dries, take a long, warm shower and wash off the clay.

To reduce the heat and inflammation of the area, apply compresses steeped in witch hazel extract.

Corn silk stripped from an ear of fresh corn is usually used as a diuretic, but it also can reduce the heat and inflammation of the testicles. Place the fresh corn silk in a clean cloth and apply directly to the testicle.

The famed early-twentieth-century herbalist-physician Dr. William Fernie observed that infinitesimal amounts of *Pulsatilla* (wood anemone) could successfully reduce swollen testicles. Place a few drops of *Pulsatilla* tincture in a tablespoon of water and apply to the testicles every few hours. "It will soon relieve a swollen testicle," said Dr. Fernie.

WATER HEALING FOR WOMEN

BREAST ABSCESS (MASTITIS)

A breast abscess starts with a mild inflammation and swelling in the breasts and armpits. The inflammation often emerges after delivery, during the nursing or weaning periods. It is crucial to treat an inflammation immediately before it becomes an abscess. *See your attending physician immediately* if the home treatments do not work quickly enough.

Breast-feeding: Whenever possible avoid antibiotic treatment.

General Information

Despite the mastitis, breast-feed your infant every 2 to 3 hours. Start each feeding with the infected breast. Continue the feeding until the breast feels soft. To alleviate pain, loosen the milk ducts, eject infectious material, and revive the milk flow, gently stroke the breast from the edge toward the nipple. Use a clean cotton or flannel cloth. To ensure that the milk ducts empty completely, gently massage the painful area while you breast-feed. To decrease stress on the nipple, change feeding positions often. To avoid cracked nipples, make sure the baby is sucking both the nipple tip as well as the darkened circle (areola) around it. Toughen the nipples by air-drying them after each feeding.

You can feed the infant 1 teaspoon of pure room-temperature water before breast-feeding. This dilutes the milk, promotes emulsion of fats, and supplies the baby with additional mineral salts.

Water and Herbal Therapy

To avoid dehydration and to offset any fever, increase your daily intake of fresh, pure water by several glasses each day.

To decrease the pain, at any time, but especially before each feeding, apply either warm water or a warm wet washcloth to the breast. To control the infection, it is useful to add either 16 drops of echinacea tincture or a quarter-teaspoon of goldenseal to the warm water. Try alternating an occasional ice pack with the warm compress.

To prevent the infection from coming back, wash your hands and nipples carefully before feeding the infant. Add drops of diluted goldenseal solution or diluted echinacea solution to the hand wash.

Caked Breasts: Apply strong peppermint tea compresses to the breasts.

Hard Breasts: Apply a mash of wet parsley leaves directly to the breasts, or in a cloth. Alternate with a wet mash of thyme leaves.

INFLAMED BREASTS

Dissolve several homeopathic arnica 6x pills in hot water. Apply warm on cotton or flannel cloths to the breasts. Alternate with compresses dipped in echinacea tincture solution. Gypsies apply chewed mallow leaves directly to the breasts to reduce inflammation. If leaves are not available, create a mallow solution by adding 16 drops of mallow tincture to a glass of warm water. Soak a flannel or soft cotton cloth in the water and apply to the breasts. To prevent inflammation and keep the breasts soft and the nipples supple and uncracked, oil the breasts and the nipples several times a week with St. John's wort or calendula oil. If the nipple is cracked or hurts, apply calendula ointment, aloe vera gel (from the leaf of the house plant), or vitamin A and D ointment.

Before you start weaning, obtain lovage tincture. Add 16 drops of the tincture to a half glass of water and rub the breasts with the solution. Also drink a cup of lovage tea (add 16 drops of lovage tincture to boiling water). It is useful to drink sage tea through the weaning process. The homeopathic cell salt (or tissue salt) natrum sulph. 6x helps to reduce breast milk.

General Therapy

Fight the internal infection in one or all of these three ways.

1. Use garlic in food or take two to three deodorized garlic capsules as a safe and strong antibactericide.
2. Add the two infection-fighter vitamins, vitamin C (as ascorbic acid powder or in ester form) and vitamin A in emulsion form, to help fight the internal infection. Holistic physicians use high doses of these vitamins to clear internal infections. *Vitamin C:* Take 2,000 mg up to 3,000 mg (depending on bowel tolerance) spaced out during the day. *Vitamin A:* Fresh carrot juice contains about 18,000 IU of vitamin A per glass. Try 1½ glasses, or start with a 25,000 IU dose of tablets for a few days. During an emergency such as this, holistic physicians work upwards to 50,000 IU and higher. In addition take a B-complex 50, 30 mg of zinc to act as a protection against future attacks, 400 IU of vitamin E, 1 tablespoon of liquid chlorophyll twice a day to purify the system, and 50 mg coenzyme Q10 each day to increase oxygen and enhance the immune system.
3. Cell salts: Dissolve 5 tablespoons ferrum phos. 6x under the tongue at the first indication of an oncoming abscess or boil. Continue until the inflammation abates.

CHILDBIRTH

Water Therapy

Drink copious quantities of red raspberry leaf tea before, during, and after giving birth. This tea helps to overcome many bleeding problems and also alleviates thirst.

If the birth is to take place at home, apply short or prolonged cold compresses to the breasts. Showers directed to the breasts can, when needed, cause vigorous contractions of the uterus.

Short cold footbaths also act via reflex on the abdominal, pelvic, and head regions, stimulating them and increasing circulation. This causes contractions in the uterus. Do not use these footbaths in the early stages of pregnancy.

To relax the uterine tissues while giving birth, apply hot moist compresses over the pubic area and the area between the vagina and anus.

In the early stages of labor, to mollify pain and promote relaxation, take a warm deep sit bath.

Two days after delivery, a hot dry pack can be applied to the breasts to encourage perspiration and help bring on the milk. Also, hot apple cider vinegar and water douches can be used to soothe the vaginal area.

After the fifth day, a cold sheet pack may be placed over the abdomen and breasts to prevent any possible congestion and to lessen the possibility of the nipples cracking and caking. (Also see "Inflamed Breasts" on page 268.)

CYSTITIS

Cystitis is an acute or chronic inflammation of the bladder that usually is the result of an infection in the kidney, prostate, or urethra. The symptoms include pain or burning upon urination as well as a strong desire to urinate even when the bladder is empty.

Water Therapy

For acute attacks, use only hot treatments. Take hot shallow sit baths several times a day.

Take hot footbaths several times a day.

Add hot catnip tea to an enema to relieve spasm or constipation.

General Therapy

To prevent yeast infection, take capsules of acidophilus every day. Add a solution of acidophilus to a vaginal douche.

Drink 2 glasses of cranberry juice every day.

Drink apple cider vinegar, honey, and water mixed. Add 1 tablespoon each of vinegar and honey to every cup of hot or cold water. This helps to establish internal balance.

Eat large amounts of watermelon. Cut the red flesh into tiny pieces, and eat one piece every 10 minutes or so throughout the day. This will flush the kidneys and bladder.

Add vitamin C to the diet and drink vegetable juices. Add small amounts of parsley or corn silk tea to peppermint or chamomile tea, or make parsley soup. Other herbs that are helpful for cystitis are juniper berries, goldenrod (tea), and horsetail (tea).

MENOPAUSE

Use all possible tonic and friction procedures to increase the tone and circulation of the body.

As often as possible during the day—especially the first thing in the morning and the very last thing at night—tread in cold water. Gradually increase your tolerance to the cold. Kneel in the water, and whenever you can, briefly sit in the cold water. This will increase your energy and zest for life.

Drink calming chamomile and/or linden tea or ginseng powder tea to normalize the body. Ginseng is energizing, too.

Avoid constipation and drink two glasses of cold water upon awakening each morning.

In general, drink as much pure water as possible each day.

Night Sweating: Before going to bed, to reduce the night sweating, take either a hot, salt-water sponge bath, or add a cup of coarse salt to a full hot-water bath. While in the bath, gently massage about a half-cup of the coarse salt on the torso, arms, shoulders, thighs, and knees. The salt-glow-rub increases circulation and produces a subtle euphoria and renewed vitality. Occasionally place astringent herbs such as white oak bark or wild alum root on the sponge or in the bathwater. Simmer 1 tablespoon of the herb to 1 quart of boiling water. Steep for 20 minutes. Strain out the herb before sponging.

To reduce night sweats, drink any of the following teas during the day: sage, strawberry leaves, or powdered goldenseal (1 teaspoon to 1 pint of boiling water). Steep, strain, and serve.

General Therapy

Researchers have found that three and a half hours of exercise a week could eliminate hot flashes altogether. Exercise also helps to avert osteoporosis. Eat a healthy diet that includes a great many green vegetables, 1 to 2 tablespoons of flaxseed oil a day (this can be obtained in capsules), and phytoestrogens such as soy products. Also make sure the diet contains sufficient fiber to avoid constipation. Control the heat from hot flashes by eating gingerroot tea or crystallized candied ginger with the sugar soaked off. Take a potent multivitamin and a balanced mineral free of sugar, yeast, and filler.

Menopausal women need supplements with vitamin E, B complex, high vitamin C, calcium, and magnesium. Some studies show that many menopausal women reported relief from hot flashes two days after starting 800 IU of vitamin E. The dose was lowered to 400 IU as soon as the flashes subsided. Vitamin E will also heal vaginal dryness and atrophy in 50 percent of the women who take it. Dr. Susan Lark of Northwestern University Medical School advises her patients not to binge on sugar, caffeine, or alcohol, as these products can trigger yeast infections and promote an overgrowth of candida.

Avoid very hot meals, heavy meals, spicy foods, and processed and refined carbohydrate foods. Hot flashes and other menopausal symptoms tend to be uncommon in vegetarian cultures that include soybeans, legumes, and black beans in the diet. Soy can also be obtained in soy flour, tofu, tempeh, and miso. Health food stores carry soy burgers, soy hot dogs, soy cheeses, and soy desserts. Fennel is also high in phytoestrogens. Celery, parsley, clover sprouts, nuts and seeds, and flaxseed oil are other foods that are useful for their estrogenic content. Herbs with estrogenic content are available in various herbal formulas such as Nature's Way Change-O-Life, Enzymatic Therapy's Femtrol, and Nature's Herbs Femchange. Most are taken three times a day.

MENSTRUAL PROBLEMS

PAINFUL PERIOD (DYSMENORRHEA)

Water Therapy

To Prevent a Painful Period: Constipation is one possible cause of a painful and/or profuse period. It can be avoided by drinking copious amounts of water during the day, and by starting each day with 2 glasses of room-temperature cold water.

Every day for several months irrigate the colon with an enema in the knee-to-chest position. This posture is soothing, and may eventually help to normalize the situation.

Take a brief hot shallow bath every day for a week before the period and 2 to 3 times a day on the first day of the period. Splash with cooler water as you end the bath. Continue this procedure for several months until a normal, pain-free period is achieved. Also between periods, take occasional alternate hot and cold sitz baths in 6 to 8 inches of water. Always end with the cold application. In addition, strengthen the body with occasional cold sponging and cold showers.

When PMS (premenstrual syndrome) is a problem, take a long cool sitz bath in 6 inches of water several times a month.

For Pain: Menstrual spasms are distressing and painful. Although heat tends to increase some of the flow, who can resist its comfort and relief? Among the hot applications are warm to hot showers directed on the lower back or hot, moist compresses applied to the spine and/or abdomen. And what can feel better after a long, nagging day of cramps than the total relaxation garnered from a full immersion in warm-to-hot water containing pine oil extracts or calming drops of valerian tincture? Olbas oil or white Tiger Balm ointment can also be massaged on the lower back area to bring blood to its surface and to alleviate pain. When ready for bed, apply a half-full hot water bottle to the area of the pain, which will ease going to sleep.

Sipping hot herbal teas also eases pain. Hot chamomile tea eases spasms and is a blessed relief for women who have painful periods. Peppermint and linden are pleasant teas at this time of the month, as is ginger tea because it also assuages digestive unease or nausea. Blueberry tea calms the system as does raspberry leaf tea. Small valerian (herb) tablets will quiet and calm the system. At this time of the month many Japanese women drink Two Peony Tea, a mixture available in Asian groceries.

Sit in a cold shallow sitz bath, and immerse the feet at the same time in a pot of hot water. This unique shallow cold to the lower extremities and hot water to the feet helps to awaken the body and dislodge the congestion in the pelvic area.

An old folk remedy that still works is to roast 2 cups of rock salt or coarse salt for 15 minutes, wrap the salt in a towel, and apply to the abdomen and ovary area.

General Therapy

Clinical studies show that capsules of evening primrose oil taken throughout the month, with the dose slightly increased as the date of the period approaches, appears to promote uterine relaxation. An old English country remedy to control painful periods consists of eating vitamin A–rich grated carrot with lemon juice and olive oil. The problem with dysmenorrhea may indicate a calcarea fluor. deficiency, which can be overcome with a daily intake of 4 calcarea fluor. cell salts (tissue salts) tablets dissolved under the tongue. If this is not available, prevent cramps by taking 1 or 2 calcium tablets every hour. Several herbal essential oils are pain-easing and restorative as well. Massage the abdomen with equal parts of these oils: fennel, melissa, and eucalyptus; or relieve the pain and spasm with this combination of oils massaged on the abdomen: chamomile oil (2 drops) and 1 drop each of fennel, peppermint, and caraway oil. This mixture can also be applied on a sanitary napkin. Nutrients that help painful periods in addition to calcium are vitamin E, iron, magnesium, and especially small amounts of vitamin B_6 to discharge fluid and bloating.

PROFUSE MENSTRUAL PERIOD (MENORRHAGIA)

Water Therapy

To Prevent a Profuse Flow: Before the period starts, take frequent hot shallow sit baths, drink room-temperature cold water every morning upon arising and before breakfast, and take a series of knee-to-chest enemas during the month (to cleanse and normalize the colon).

To ensure a decrease in the expected period, just before and during the first part of the period, sit briefly in a cold shallow sit bath. This bath works even better if the feet are simultaneously placed in a hot footbath.

To Decrease a Profuse Flow: On the first day of the period, drink a half-cup of black bean juice 3 times during the day. This will eventually lessen the profuse flow.

When a menstrual flow is exceptionally heavy, either one of the following reflex cold-water remedies will help to control and decrease the menstrual flow: an ice bag between the thighs or a cold footbath in several inches of cold water.

Several herbs act as styptics and can be used internally as vaginal douches: witch hazel extract or teas made from the astringent herbs shepherd's purse, bayberry bark, and white oak bark. Of these, witch hazel extract is the easiest to purchase; it is available in pharmacies. Use the Dickinson brand over a generic brand. To use witch hazel in a douche, dilute it by adding several tablespoons of the extract to 1 pint of body-temperature warm water. Tampons can be submerged in the extract and applied internally. Depending on the extent of the flow, exchange the tampon for a fresh herb-soaked one every half-hour to two hours.

Shepherd's purse (*Capsella bursa-pastoris*) has been used for hundreds of years by European village healers to stop profuse bleeding, and unlike witch hazel, it can also be used as an antihemorrhaging drink. Add 1 tablespoon of the dried herb to a mug of boiling water. Steep, strain, and drink. Its reputation as a styptic is outstanding, and it is generally believed that 1 cup will be all that is needed. To use shepherd's purse herb in a douche, add 1 heaping tablespoon of the dried herb to 1 quart of boiling water, steep covered, strain, and apply the clear tea internally with a bulb-syringe douche. As with witch hazel, shepherd's purse can also be used internally on a tampon to subdue a profuse period.

A final word on styptics: Cayenne pepper is a surprisingly effective blood stopper. Dare to use a pinch of cayenne pepper in any restorative herbal tea.

General Therapy

Heavy or profuse bleeding during the menstrual cycle is thought to be a temporary hormonal imbalance, possibly caused by the body's inability to properly synthesize prostaglandins. Help to rebalance the body with essential fatty acids (EFA) such as evening primrose, borage, or black currant seed oil. Although a heavy profuse menstrual flow usually causes a mild iron depletion, insufficient levels of iron in the system can also cause such a profuse flow. When supplementation of iron is needed, do it with the help of a health care practitioner who is skilled in using nutrient remedies. Meanwhile, drink orange juice for the vitamin C and folic acid content to strengthen the capillary walls, to help reduce a profuse menstrual flow, and to increase the absorption of iron in the diet. Vitamin C foods include fruits, nuts, seeds, and buckwheat. Choose a high-potency vitamin C with flavonoids and take 1,000 mg 2 times a day. Also, cook acidic foods such as tomatoes and applesauce in cast-iron pots to leach the iron from the pot into the food. Women with a profuse flow usually need vitamin A–rich foods, and should be eating some of the following each day: carrots, yams, sweet potatoes, spinach, cantaloupe, broccoli, and kale. Other antioxidant supplements are B_{12} and vitamin E, which may also reduce endometrial bleeding by modifying free radical activity and prostaglandin action.

Studies indicate that an underactive thyroid contributes to many menstrual problems. Medical nutritionists sometimes prescribe minute amounts of thyroid to control a profuse flow and other menstrual irregularities.

SCANTY OR DELAYED MENSTRUATION (AMENORRHEA)

Lack of a period is due to faulty blood supply, which in turn may be due to a number of other causes.

Water Therapy

Copious amounts of fresh water and a daily enema before sleep will stimulate more normal menstrual activity.

Avoid constipation by drinking 2 glasses of room-temperature cold water upon arising each day.

As a general procedure, take frequent hot sitz baths at various times of the day. Also take hot full baths before going to bed each night.

Several days before the period is expected, drink hot herbal teas such as rosemary, sage, chamomile, lady's mantle, or lemon verbena to stimulate the onset of the period. Other kitchen herbs are helpful in overcoming a delayed period, such as basil leaves, melissa or lemon balm, thyme leaves, fennel plant, or dill leaves.

Several days before the period is expected utilize any of these alternate hot and cold techniques: Immerse the lower extremities in alternate hot and cold shallow sitz baths; irrigate the vaginal region with alternate hot and cold douches; and apply alternate hot and cold compresses to the pelvic area.

Along with the above alternate treatments occasionally use these hot-water applications: Apply prolonged hot moist compresses to the pelvic area. Take at least one hot shallow sitz bath. When in bed keep your feet warm by applying a hot water bottle.

In cases of delayed period because of nervousness, frequently sponge or immerse hands, feet, breasts, and abdomen in cold water. Calming teas can be used to allay nervousness. Once your nerves are calmed, the period often starts again. Valerian tablets are quieting, calming, and extremely helpful in overcoming nervousness. Drink chamomile flower tea, and apply a hot chamomile flower poultice to the groin and lower back area. Also drink linden tea.

German herbalist-physicians often use hedge hyssop (*Gratiola officinalis*) to induce a delayed menstrual period. Combine 1 tablespoon of each of the following to 1 quart of boiling water, steep for 20 minutes, and take on an empty stomach 1 hour before breakfast: hedge hyssop herb, rue leaf, senna leaf, and fennel fruit. This combination can also be prepared for you by a compounding pharmacist with equal amounts of the above herbs. Dr. Rudolf Fritz Weiss in *Lehrbuch der Phytotherapie* speaks well of this formula but warns that rue (*Ruta graveolens*), while calming and sedative, as well as helpful in overcoming an absence of menstrual flow, can be dangerous if the delayed period is due to a pregnancy, because it may cause a spontaneous miscarriage.

General Therapy

For most of the month until the period arrives, take 1 kelp tablet in the morning and another one at noon (never in the evening) to normalize the menstrual flow. Pineapple, figs, and papaya fruits contain special enzymes believed to be helpful in overcoming a delayed, suppressed, or scanty period. Gingerroot candy and gingerroot tea are also helpful.

PREGNANCY

Water Therapy

Drink water freely to stimulate the kidneys. Especially drink 2 glasses of cold water every morning before breakfast. After this, gently massage the abdomen for 5 minutes. Continue this throughout the pregnancy; it will help to regulate the bowels.

Take a warm-water shallow bath for 30 minutes every day, at noon, whenever possible. This helps drain the veins by osmosis and prevent and correct varicose veins.

The easiest method of cleansing during the last stages of pregnancy is to stand in several inches of warm water and take a cool shower.

If there is albumen in the urine, or serious vertigo or dizziness, use a hot dry pack every second or third night. After the sixth month of pregnancy, try to develop a weekly sweating routine. Drink a large glass of hot lemonade with honey. Then get into bed, place several hot water bottles on your feet and sides, and envelop yourself in blankets. After an hour the bottles can be taken away and you can sleep for the rest of the night. If you prefer, you may get up to cool off your body with a tepid sponging, change your bedclothes, and go back to bed to sleep. This weekly process will help eliminate waste materials and relieve the overstrained circulation of the abdominal and pelvic organs.

To avoid a miscarriage, take frequent 2-second cold half-baths.

Hot Tubs and Pregnancy: Pregnant women should not go into hot tubs. They must avoid high heat during the first months of pregnancy. High heat, even high fever, can cause brain-damage to the fetus.

Pregnancy Cramps: Add calcium and B_6 to the diet.

OTHER PELVIC AREA PROBLEMS

SPASMS IN BLADDER, RECTUM, AND UTERUS

Apply prolonged hot moist compresses to the pelvic area to relax the muscles of the bladder, rectum, and uterus. This relieves spasms in these organs and increases menstrual flow. To decrease the flow, sit in a cold shallow bath.

Showers on the shoulder area act by reflex on the pelvic area.

PELVIC CRAMPS DUE TO PERIOD

Sit in a cold shallow bath. At the same time, immerse the feet in a hot footbath.

PELVIC INFLAMMATION

Sit in a cold shallow bath. At the same time, immerse the feet in a hot footbath.

PELVIC CONGESTION

Take a hot footbath.

NONINFLAMMATORY PELVIC PROBLEMS

Sit in a hot shallow bath or immerse the feet in a hot footbath.

UTERINE HEMORRHAGE

Apply a cold compress to the inner thighs, vagina, the area between the vagina and anus, and the lower back.

UTERINE CONGESTION

Direct a prolonged, cold, low-pressure fan shower to the chest.

UTERINE INFLAMMATION

Sit on a stool in the bathtub, separate your knees, and direct a cold, low-pressure fan shower to the area from the navel to the pubic bone. This cold action contracts the uterus, reduces inflammation, and acts on the bladder, uterus, and ovaries via reflex action.

BLADDER, BOWELS, AND UTERUS

Short applications to abdomen, hands, or feet cause contractions of the muscles.

VAGINAL PROBLEMS

VAGINITIS

Vaginitis is a somewhat umbrella diagnosis with a variety of discharges. Consult a physician to determine the kind of discharge. Once this has been determined, it will be possible to decide on the proper remedy.

The vagina has a normal population of protective lactobacillus. To restore colonies of this valuable microorganism, each day:

1. Drink a half-teaspoon of any potent, powdered lactobacillus in a quarter-cup of water (or swallow a capsule containing the product).
2. Create a solution with 1 tablespoon of powdered lactobacillus to a half-cup of water. Soak a tampon in the solution. Apply internally for several hours. Repeat again during the day. Continue the drink and insertion of the tampon for several weeks.

Three times a week take a tepid-water sitz bath for half an hour. Or, add an ounce of pine extract, strong thyme tea, thyme extract, chamomile extract, or chamomile tea. To relieve and overcome most cases of vaginitis, Japanese healers commonly add an umeboshi plum to this sitz bath and hold part of the plum to the vaginal area.

The trichomonas organism grows in an alkaline environment. Acidify the area with douches of apple cider vinegar. Otherwise take douches with either tea tree oil or betadine. On occasion, trichomonas infections are caused by accidentally leaving in the vagina a foreign object such as a tampon, sponge, diaphragm, or pessary.

If there is burning or itching take a tepid-temperature sitz bath to which a cup of apple cider vinegar or a cup of blended or colloidal oatmeal (Aveeno) has been added.

Douching: Despite the barrage of advertisements to the contrary, current researchers warn women, especially of childbearing age, to be wary of chemical douches. Recent reports indicate that too much douching has been associated with life-threatening tubal (ectopic) pregnancies.

VAGINAL SPASMS

Douche with hot water or hot rosemary tea to relieve the pain and irritation of the spasm. The hot irrigation increases the absorption of inflammatory cellular fluid.

VAGINAL CONGESTION

Douche with tepid (90°F) water or weak rosemary tea for up to 30 minutes. Avoid very cold or very hot douches during pregnancy. Cold douches can cause contractions in the uterus.

VAGINISMUS (PAINFUL SPASM OF THE VAGINA)

Douche with hot water and take hot shallow sit baths and frequent hot footbaths. Rosemary tea or chamomile tea may be added to the water.

For additional relief, occasionally apply ice wrapped in a towel from the shoulder region of the spine to the neck.

CANDIDIASIS (YEAST INFECTION)

Water Therapy

Douche with acidophilus yogurt or dissolved acidophilus tablets or powder in water for 5 consecutive nights. You can also add 4 drops of tea tree oil to a douche (or combine 4 drops of tea tree oil and 4 tablespoons of almond, olive, safflower, or sesame oil and apply with a tampon). Other effective douches are slippery elm, thyme, or goldenseal tea plus 2 tablespoons of witch hazel extract to soothe the symptoms of itching and burning associated with a yeast infection.

For 3 days in a row steep in a 10- to 15-minute hip (sitz) bath to sooth and heal the area. It is useful to insert an acidophilus tampon prior to the bath.

Restore helpful bacteria to the colon with an enema containing acidophilus culture.

General Therapy

Take 3 to 5 tablets of natrum phos. 6x cell salt (or tissue salt) under the tongue 3 times a day to relieve pain and itching.

WATER HEALING FOR CHILDREN

BAD-TASTING MEDICINE

Many children resist taking liquid medicine. Let the child suck on an ice cube first to numb the mouth, then give the medicine. Another method is to crush ice, put the medicine in the crushed ice, and let the child suck on the ice.

BEDWETTING

See Part 3.

BOILS

Massage ice on the first indication of a boil to halt it.

CHICKENPOX

Water Therapy

Think of water as an all-purpose, safe remedy to flush the system, hydrate the cells, cleanse the skin, and relieve itching.

To maintain cleanliness and relieve itching, give the child several warm baths a day with Aveeno, a colloidal oatmeal milled into a fine powder. It is available in drugstores. Once this bath treatment is dispersed into the bathwater, it helps to relieve itchy, sore skin. During the bath, protect the child from drafts.

Use a child's size bulb enema to flush the bowel area.

Give water, raspberry, or fennel tea or diluted orange juice throughout the day. Maintain a liquid diet as long as there is fever. When the fever subsides, give the child an all-fruit diet for one day.

General Therapy

Investigate the use of cell (tissue salts) therapy to control the fever and deal with the eruptions. To further relieve itching and promote drying of eruptions, liberally spray or pat on calamine lotion.

COLIC

Water Therapy

A hot shallow sit bath or a hot footbath will help to overcome stomach spasms by reflex action.

Chamomile is a very effective remedy for controlling colic in children. Make a tea by adding boiling water to the flowers. Steep, cool, and strain into a cup or a baby's bottle. It relieves stomach upsets and spasms.

General Therapy

When in doubt about severe and persistent gas pains, see a physician.

COLD SORES

At the first indication of an emerging cold sore, rub an ice cube on the area. If you catch it right away, you will halt the eruption. (For more, see Part 3.)

CONGESTION

If your child has a congested nose, keep a steam vaporizer going in her or his room. If you don't have a vaporizer (get one soon!), turn your bathroom into a sauna by closing the door and turning on the hot water in the shower (close the curtains so the child won't get splashed). Wrap up your ailing, congested child and let him or her sit in the steamy bathroom for five minutes or so. Steam unclogs those nasal and sinus passages.

CONSTIPATION

See Part 3.

CONVULSIONS

Water Therapy

Use the warm pack, or a modified cold wrap. Place a long cotton nightgown on the child. Dip the child and nightgown briefly into cold water in the bathtub, and then quickly wrap the child in an old flannel or wool blanket. Place the child in bed and cover him or her with a light blanket or feather cover. Repeat the procedure several times, if necessary.

CRYING SPELL

Water Therapy

Do you want to see magic? Gently place a fitful child in a warm bath, and the crying should stop. This can be done any time of the day or night.

Add linden or chamomile tea to the drinking water or bottle. This will help to overcome spasms and trapped gas. If there doesn't seem to be a reason for the crying, apply the wet cold abdominal compress, and cover with a flannel blanket. This technique is highly successful. Repeat twice a day until the crying spells stop.

General Therapy

The water remedies work either to alleviate spasms, or totally alter body imbalance. You can also use the Bach Flower Remedies. Place 2 drops of Bach walnut flowers or 2 drops of Bach chicory flowers in a small amount of water. Have the child drink the preparation. These nontoxic flower infusions will also work on tearful adults.

CUTS

First wash the cut. To soften the emotional effect of blood flowing, try to use a red washcloth. Apply calendula lotion, the pure juice of pot marigold (*Succus calendula* or *Calendula officinalis*) as homeopathy, or Dickinson's triple distilled witch hazel extract to stop the bleeding from cuts.

DIARRHEA

Water Therapy

Prevent dehydration by letting the child suck on crushed ice. For diarrhea, in addition to giving the child small teaspoons of pure Coca-Cola syrup (or Classic Coke) to cure the diarrhea, add teaspoons of the syrup to pure water and freeze as ice cubes. Crush the ice cubes, or place in a clean washcloth so that they can be sucked.

DIPHTHERIA

The following water therapies were used by physician-hydrotherapists before the creation of antibiotics. If there is an outbreak of this disease, use these therapies until your physician can be reached.

Water Therapy

Snugly wrap the child's neck in a damp cold-water compress or a diluted apple cider vinegar compress. Replace it as soon as it is hot, every 15 minutes or so. For body wrapping, use a long cotton nightgown or two pinned hand towels or bath towels. Dip the towels or nightgown into a mixture of half apple cider vinegar and half water, wring it out so that it is still damp, and wrap it around the child from the armpits to the knees. Pin it in place. Cover the child with bedclothes. Change the wrapping every 15 minutes until the body heat decreases. The child should also drink copious amounts of water and pineapple juice. Pineapple juice seems to be helpful in detaching the membrane on the throat.

Several Times a Day: Flush out the colon with an enema. Use a vaporizer in the room with pineapple juice in the water. Apply cold sectional sponging every 3 to 4 hours to stimulate the nervous system and the heart. If there is numbness in the body, apply a hot moist compress on the affected nerves for 20 minutes. Follow each hot application with a cold sponging and swift drying of the area. Do not allow drafts in the room.

Between Treatments: Apply a cold compress to the heart area. This acts as a tonic.

Threat of Suffocation: Place the child in a full hot bath for 1 to 20 minutes. At the same time use cold water to sponge the back of the neck, the entire back, the shoulders, and spine area.

Dr. Kuhn of Germany has experimented with an ice-water spray over the membrane of the throat. This helps to loosen the membrane. If the patient cooperates and expectorates as soon as the water touches the throat, the throat can be cleared. Repeat every half-hour.

DIZZINESS

Water Therapy

Dizziness may be due to sluggishness of the liver. The child should drink 2 glasses of cold water a half-hour before breakfast.

Take a towel dipped in half apple cider vinegar and half cold water, and wind it around the child from the armpits to the knees, several times a day, for 1 hour at a time.

EAR INFECTIONS

See Part 3.

ECZEMA

See Part 3.

ERUPTIONS

Water Therapy

Bacterial Infections: If there is a threat of scarlet fever or measles, or any bacterial epidemic, bring out the eruptions and toxins in this way: Wash the child with a mild salt solution, or wrap the child in a towel or shirt dipped in a solution of salt. Wrap the child in blankets, put him or her to bed, and cover lightly with bedclothes. The eruptions will soon be visible. Have the child drink lots of water.

This therapy should not be used in lieu of consulting a physician.

Nonbacterial Eruptions: Apply shirts or towels that have been dipped in hayflower tea before bedtime every other day for 2 weeks. This will bring out the eruptions and toxins. Have the child drink lots of water.

In both cases, strengthen the child with frequent cold baths or cold spongings, but never allow the child to become chilled!

GERMAN MEASLES

Rubella, or German measles, is a mild form of measles that usually lasts three days. Symptoms are a mild fever, a sore throat, and a red rash that starts on the head and moves to the trunk and limbs.

Water Therapy

The child should be urged to drink water constantly because this quickly reduces the fever and encourages the ejection of toxins.

Sponge the child throughout the day with warm water.

If itching is a problem, briefly place the child in a warm bath containing Aveeno, a colloidal oatmeal found in drugstores.

HERNIA

Water Therapy

Kneipp used the following water therapies for children's hernia. Wrap the child in a towel dipped in fresh pine extract and neutral to cold water. Cover the area from the armpits to the knees. Apply for 1½ hours.

Alternate this treatment with 1 hour applications of a neutral compress that has been dipped in hayflower tea to the stomach area.

Once a day, wash the child in cold water.

To strengthen the child, each day for a week direct a mild stream of water to different areas of the body. Concentrate on only one area at a time. Start with showers to the upper part of the back, then sponge the entire body. Toward the end of the week sit the child in several inches of cold water for a few seconds. After this, start the child walking in cold water as often as possible. Occasionally direct a mild stream of water to the knee area.

Check with your physician or pediatrician. *This water therapy treatment does not replace their medical attention and supervision.*

HEAT REACTION

See Part 3.

MASTOIDITIS

Mastoiditis is an acute or chronic inflammation of bone and cells of the mastoid—the area behind the ear lobe. It is usually the direct result of a middle ear infection.

See a physician immediately. Use water therapy only in an emergency.

Water Therapy

Older Children and Adults: The following water therapy relieves the pain by inhibiting the flow of blood in the mastoid, and by diverting blood from the inflamed area.

Apply a moist hot compress to the mastoid bone. At the same time, take a hot leg bath and place an ice bag on the carotid artery (on the neck) on the same side as the pain.

Continue the treatment for 20 to 30 minutes, up to an hour.

Follow this treatment with a cold, vigorous friction massage of the limbs and trunk of the body.

MEASLES

Water Therapy

Water is essential for bringing down fever and avoiding dehydration. Give babies at least a spoonful of water every half-hour. Follow the thirst instincts of toddlers and older children by giving them as much water as requested, or if not requested, as much water as they will tolerate. To reduce the patient's internal heat, dissolve some gingersnaps in water, or make a diluted ginger tea and add to some of the drinks during the day. Other appropriate and helpful fluids include raspberry leaf tea, fennel seed or lemon balm (melissa) tea, and clear chicken or vegetable broth. The patient will also benefit from small amounts of orange, grape, or carrot juice.

Reduce itching with a series of oatmeal baths. Either grind regular oatmeal into smaller particles, or better still, purchase Aveeno, the prepared colloidal oatmeal that dissolves instantly in bathwater.

The rural people of Great Britain still use calendula (marigold) tea as a tonic drink, to expedite the release of the eruptions and speed up the healing time of the disease.

If the patient is fidgety or restless, give him or her chamomile tea or a tablet of homeopathic chamomilla, once or twice a day.

Sebastian Kneipp, the Bavarian master herbalist who codified all the known water therapies in the late nineteenth century, advised using hayflower "dips" to detoxify the child. Hayflowers were readily available to rural populations at that time. Now you can obtain Biokosma's superb Hayflower Bath (extract). The double hayflower compress acts as a magnet to draw out internal impurities and brings eruptions to the surface of the skin. Add 2 tablespoons of the brown extract to a large pot of boiled water. Plunge a cotton shirt a size or two larger than the patient into the bath, wring it out, and, as it will have lost its intense heat by this time, place it on the child. Immediately wrap the child in a cotton or wool blanket and put her or him to bed. The double wrap—the wet shirt and enveloping dry blanket, which doesn't allow air to get to the wet surface—encourages perspiration and hastens the emergence of eruptions. This wet/dry wrap encourages the millions of pores on the skin to push the virus out of the system. Afterwards, keep the child covered with another clean sheet or cotton blanket and rinse him or her off, one area of the body at a time. The child should sleep peacefully after this experience.

Should the child develop a cough, apply a folded tepid, wet, wrung-out cloth to the chest and cover it immediately with a slightly larger, dry wool (or nonporous cotton) cloth or blanket. No air should be allowed to penetrate to the wet compress. The body responds to the cold by forcing blood to circulate in the abdominal area, and the dry wool covering on the chest forces an internal flow of blood to the area. The congestion should break up from within.

General Therapy

For the duration of the measles, shield the child from bright light to make her or him feel more comfortable. Keep the room well ventilated but draw the shades to keep the room light dim.

Echinacea is a potent antiviral. Use child-sized dosages to support the healing process and immune system function. As soon as the child's tongue is clear and the temperature is reduced, give an all-fruit cleansing diet for several days. To prevent secondary infections for several weeks afterwards, give the patient child-sized doses of vitamin C, zinc, and beta-carotene (for vitamin A) to support the healing process and to strengthen the immune system. Do not exceed suggested doses.

Incubation period for the measles is 8 to 12 days from exposure to onset of symptoms, with an average interval of 14 days to appearance of rash. Period of communicability is 1 to 2 days before the onset of symptoms, or 3 to 5 days before the appearance of rash until 4 days after rash appearance. Children should be excluded from school at least 4 days after the onset of rash.

For German measles, the incubation period is 16 to 18 days, with outside limits of 14 to 21 days. Period of communicability is one week before until 5 to 7 days after onset of rash. Children should be excluded from school for 7 days after onset of rash.

MUMPS

Isolate the child until the swelling goes down. It usually takes 8 days for the child to resume normal activity. The incubation period for mumps is 17 or 18 days.

Water Therapy

To inhibit the spread of the infection, apply an ice compress over the swelling for several minutes every 10 minutes.

To alleviate both pain and sensitivity, alternate 15-minute wet, moist warm and 5-minute cool compresses to the area of the swelling. Add rosemary to the compresses to increase circulation.

Hot castor oil packs placed on the swollen area will also ease the pain of mumps. Gently heat deodorized castor oil like the pure Palma Christi. Submerge soft cotton or flannel cloths in the heated castor oil, wring out, and place warm on the swollen glands. This warming and healing application may be repeated as often as required during the day.

Reduce the fever by having the child drink copious amounts of fluids, including a tranquilizing chamomile tea several times a day. When the fever abates apply hot, moist applications to the swellings.

To help the child feel more comfortable and fall asleep, select a large cotton scarf and wind it across the head, past the swollen glands, and around the neck. Don't make it too tight, but protect the area from air and drafts. The warmth of the winding makes most children feel comfortable, but don't insist on the arrangement if the child doesn't like it.

Should a boy complain of testicular pain, apply ice packs to the thighs and the general region. Improvise a small-sized "jock strap" to support the scrotum. This is a time when all the youngsters need complete bed rest, but rest is particularly important for boys since this virus can impair their future fertility. Should a boy be restless, fidgety, or superactive, explain the situation to him and improvise quiet games and reading experiences. Calmness and quiet are essential for this period.

Headaches may be a problem and may range from minor to splitting ordeals. Damp compresses of peppermint tea are pleasant and help to ease the headaches. It also helps to thoroughly relax the eyes by applying room-temperature slices of cucumber, or witch hazel compresses to closed eyelids. (Also read "Headaches" in Part 3.)

General Therapy

Bolster the child's immune function with child-sized doses of echinacea drops, which are to be given in tiny doses throughout the day. Never use echinacea for more than 10 days at a time—take a 10-day rest and start again.

NIGHTMARE ZAP

Create an instant monster zap machine. Into a plastic spray bottle pour fresh water, green or blue vegetable coloring, and some wonderful spice extract such as vanilla, cinnamon, or nutmeg, because monsters don't like that good smell. You and your child, or if old enough, your child alone, sprays under the bed, around the bed, and in the closet until all the bogeymen are named and routed.

SCARLET FEVER

Water Therapy

Give the child plenty of hot liquids and fruit juices. At the beginning of the treatment, give the child a little cinnamon bark tea every hour. Later, give the tea every 2 hours until the temperature drops. Also use this tea as a gargle.

Salt Shirts: Add several handfuls of coarse or regular salt to 1 quart of cold water. Dip a long shirt into the salt solution. Place it on the child. Cover the child with a warm blanket for 1 hour. Change the shirt to a dry one, and again put the child to bed. The second shirt will bring out the eruptions. If necessary, the salt shirt may be used for a third time. This will bring out any remaining internal toxins.

Instead of the salt-dipped shirt, you can use salt washings. After the washing, do not dry the child but put him or her to bed wet under light covers. If the child becomes overheated, sponge the entire body. At the onset of the disease, wash the child every half hour. Later, wash every 2 to 3 hours; eventually, wash once or twice a day.

This series of water therapies will bring this difficult infection to a close in only a few days.

If it is not possible to use the salt spongings or salt shirts, use other perspiration-inducing techniques such as hot baths or hot blanket packs. Apply a cold compress on the forehead during these hot treatments.

If the child becomes comatose, place him or her in a warm bath and rub the spine with ice, or wash the child in sections with hot water and a sponge. Use 3 swift spongings to each series, and repeat the series 4 times a day. In between treatments, apply a cold compress to the forehead and renew every 20 minutes.

If the throat needs to be relaxed, apply alternate 10-minute hot moist compresses and 5-minute cold compresses.

If there is some heart complication, apply a cold compress to the heart area every 15 minutes.

Keep up the warm bath every morning for a week after the crisis has passed. Make sure the child is never chilled.

Water therapy, however, does not replace the need for proper medical care of scarlet fever.

General Therapy

There is usually a 3- to 7-day incubation period, a week of isolation, and then the patient returns to normal. The use of water therapy can greatly expedite the healing process.

SLEEPLESSNESS

If the baby can't get to sleep, prepare a warm bath and let the child soak for a few minutes. Wrap the child in a large towel, put on pajamas, cover with light blanket. According to the journal of the American Sleep Disorders Association, the warm bath raises the core body temperature; and the "compensatory cooling down afterwards helps deepen sleep."

STOMACHACHES

Dilute your favorite herbal teas such as chamomile (unless the child has hayfever), peppermint, linden, or fennel. Give half water, half herbal tea.

STRENGTHENING FOR CHILDREN

Accustom your child to cold-water applications. End every warm bath with a few seconds of a cold-water splash. Work up to a few seconds of just cold water. Later show your child how to walk or stand in cold running water in the bathtub. Keep strict safety precautions by holding on to a bar rail. Cold dips and walking in cold water will have a positive lifelong impact on your child's good health.

TEETHING

Water Therapy

Wet stockings work by diverting pain and congestion from the mouth. Have ready 1 pair of long cotton stockings or 2 strips of cotton fabric, 1 pair of long wool stockings or 2 soft wool scarves, and a pan of cold water. Dip the cotton stockings into cold water, wring out thoroughly, and put them on the child's feet. If using cotton strips, wet them, wring out, and wrap the legs. Immediately place the wool wrappings or wool socks over the cold, wet stockings. This alerts the child's internal temperature regulation mechanism to warm the cold area with fresh blood, temporarily diverting the blood away from the upper areas of the body. When this happens it dulls the sense of pain from the teething and the mind is also lulled into blessed torpor and sleep. All these things should occur consecutively. If for some reason the child's feet are not quickly warmed with this technique, take off the compresses and briskly rub the feet dry.

General Therapy

The child can suck on peeled semisweet pieces of apple, oven-dried wheat crusts, or orris root (available in health food stores). The following herbs can be diluted and applied to the gums: 1 drop of vanilla extract plus olive oil; 1 drop of clove oil plus olive oil; or 1 drop of peppermint oil plus olive oil.

Avoid giving your child a bottle of milk, fruit juice, or other sweetened liquids as a pacifier or comforter. According to the American Dental Association, decay occurs when sweetened liquids are given and are left clinging to an infant's teeth for long periods of time. Many sweet liquids cause problems, including milk, formula, and fruit juice. Bacteria in the mouth use these sugars as food, then produce acids that attack the teeth. Each time your child drinks these liquids, acids attack for twenty minutes longer. After many attacks, the teeth can decay.

part 5
Water Healing, Sports, and Exercise

Vigorous exercise dulls the body's ability to gauge thirst, so do not use thirst as a guide for drinking fluids while exercising. To prevent dehydration, cramps, headaches, or lack of coordination, exercisers should drink about 2 cups of cold water about 15 minutes before exercising, and about a half to a whole cup every 15 minutes thereafter. Cold drinks are more effective because they leave the stomach more quickly than warm drinks.

Dr. Norman Shealy offers this water intake formula to meet your daily water requirements and maintain your saliva and urine at the neutral (neither acid nor alkaline) pH of 6.4: Divide your weight by 2 to give the amount of ounces your body needs each day.

A self-test is whether you pass water several times a day, and the color of your urine, which should be a pale, whitish yellow. If you are passing infrequent amounts of dark yellow or clotted urine, you are drinking too little water. Another self-test is whether you are developing dark circles under your eyes. If the dark circles aren't from lack of sleep or unusual stress, it may well be that your body requires more water. To clear the kidneys and flush the system, kidney experts expect a patient to produce a urinary output of 2 quarts a day. This output requires drinking at least 8 glasses of drinking water.

TO PREVENT DEHYDRATION WHILE EXERCISING

How Much Water	When	Temperature
2 cups	15 minutes before exercising	Cold only
½ to 1 cup	Every 15 minutes	Cold only

The primary mechanism for maintaining normal body temperature during physical exercise is the evaporation of sweat. Athletes, especially younger athletes who exercise in the heat, are in danger of dehydration. Dehydration brings on the risk of heat cramps, heat exhaustion, and heat stroke. According to D. L. Squire at Duke University Medical Center, Durham, North Carolina, "The athlete should begin exercise well hydrated: frequent consumption of cold water during exercise decreases likelihood of significant dehydration. After exercise, the athlete should continue drinking to replace fluid losses. Cold water remains the preferred choice for fluid replacement during exercise."

What about drinking water before, during, and after outdoor activities in cold weather? In an informal poll of fifty people, most thought that they needed to drink water mainly during hot weather, hardly ever during cold weather. They are wrong. It is possible to get extremely dehydrated in cold weather. Sweating during exercise plus normal cold weather breathing in which you warm and moisturize the air you inhale produce dehydration. This makes you feel colder.

Most people are enticed to warm or hot drinks when they are cold to warm themselves up, but U.S. Army research shows that it takes about a quart of hot liquid at a time to produce even a slight elevation in body heat. The effect of the hot drink is so fleeting that one sometimes ends up feeling colder instead of warmer. The Army tells its people to drink cold water when the weather is cold because it goes through the body faster.

A report indicates that older people often forget to drink during exercise even though they may be hot and sweaty. Since the sense of thirst can fade without our realizing it, exercise experts advise older people in particular to drink whether or not they are thirsty.

Although it is always a good idea to drink as much water as possible, some long-distance runners and ultramarathoners have developed hyponatremia (a rare but potentially fatal condition), which is an abnormally low concentration of sodium in the blood. Overdrinking increases the risk of developing this condition by diluting blood sodium. Symptoms include nausea, vomiting, muscle weakness, headache, and disorientation, as well as bloating and puffiness in the face and fingers.

According to Susan Gilbert in the *New York Times,* Dr. William Roberts, a spokesman for the American College of Sports Medicine, suggests that runner calculate their "sweat rate" ahead of time to find out how much water they should be drinking. To calculate your "sweat rate," weigh yourself, exercise for half an hour at the pace and conditions you will be racing in, then weigh yourself again to find out how many pounds you've lost through perspiration. For every pound that you lost, you should drink a pint of water per hour during the race.

Sports drinks that contain carbohydrates and electrolytes, such as Gatorade, can also replace sodium lost through perspiration. Another way to ensure proper blood sodium concentration if you are a runner is to salt your food in the days approaching an upcoming race.

Patients with known high blood pressure often take diuretics to increase their water loss. Oddly, the water loss may be too high in some cases and might lead to minor dehydration. It is advisable to check with your doctor to make certain your fluid intake is adequate and appropriate. Some people, many of them older folks, don't feel thirsty during the day. Our signals on thirst diminish when we get older, so don't trust them to tell you when you need to drink. Too little fluid in the system leads to low blood volume, which in turn can contribute to low blood pressure. If you've been told you have low blood pressure, make sure you have an adequate fluid intake. People with low blood pressure sometimes feel woozy and faint when they stand up. To encourage a stronger heart rate and overcome the dizziness, it helps to quickly stretch, yawn, and take deep breaths.

EXERCISE RECOVERY

Water Therapy

Take cayenne pepper (¼ teaspoon in 1 cup of hot water) before stretching to increase circulation, raise body temperature, and help muscle flexibility.

Very short hot applications of water or very brief hot baths are the best means of quickly recovering from exercise exhaustion. Long hot applications or long hot baths will cause muscular weakness. Always end the hot-water applications with a toning cold-water splash.

Each evening before bedtime, tread in cold water for several minutes. This strengthens the body and prevents postexercise leg cramps.

Hot ginger baths will help to relax stiff muscles. Dissolve small amounts of ginger powder in boiling water and add to the hot bath. Gradually increase the amount of ginger from 1 teaspoon to 1 tablespoon, depending on your tolerance.

ACHILLES TENDON

Water Therapy

Whirlpool therapy and plunging the feet in alternate hot and cold footbaths will increase the circulation. Treading in cold water will also strengthen the feet and help tone up the entire body. Water treatment is an adjunct to general therapy.

General Therapy

Athletes know that taping around the heel that is too tight sometimes produces a strain in the Achilles tendon. Other times, the strain is caused by one side of the body being higher than another. This imbalance is easily adjusted by a professional chiropractor or osteopath. Also, a heel lift will help to balance the unequal sides of the body.

ANKLE INJURIES

WEAK ANKLES

Water Therapy

Tread in cold water as often as possible.

Frequently plunge the feet into alternate hot and cold footbaths.

SPRAIN

Water Therapy

Minor Sprain: An initial hour of ice therapy and elevation reduces swelling and tenderness. Afterward, use Gibney taping, and every several hours strap the ice bag over the taping with an elastic bandage. The ankle will need continuous elevation. Do a minimum of walking. Use a raw onion wrap over the ankle during the night to reduce pain and swelling. Apple cider vinegar wrappings are also helpful.

Major Sprain: Follow the same instructions for taping, compression, ice therapy, and elevation. Prevent further swelling and internal bleeding by bed rest. As above, raw onion or apple cider vinegar wrappings are helpful.

Rehabilitation: A hot and cold footbath, suggested by Sayers "Bud" Miller at Pennsylvania State University, is excellent rehabilitation therapy for sprains.

Note: This is one of the rare applications that ends with hot water. Most alternate applications must end with cold water, and most hot water treatments are followed by a toning with cold water.

FOREFOOT (BELOW THE ANKLE SPRAIN)

The area below the ankle is the calcaneocuboid, an area often twisted or turned in daily life and in sports.

Water Therapy

Use ice therapy immediately. Attach the ice bag with an elastic bandage to produce compression, and elevate the foot. The time required for rehabilitation depends on the age and fragility of the patient. Most athletes will be able to walk without pain within 2 to 3 days.

General Therapy

Use a figure eight strapping, and continue for 2 weeks. I like arnica lotion for such pain, and apply it directly to the pained area.

BONE BRUISE ON ANKLE

This area tends to be susceptible to bruises and will remain tender after the first bruise.

Water Therapy

Attach an ice bag, placing another fabric between the ankle and the bag. Create some compression with an elastic bandage. Elevate the ankle area.

General Therapy

Generally, keeping off your feet for 24 to 48 hours helps to heal the bruise.

In sports, it is a good practice to attach a thin rubber padding on the outside of the shoe or skate to prevent further problems. If the strainlike pain persists, some trainers tape the ankle on a routine basis.

ARCH SPASM

Water Therapy

Mild Spasm: Attach an ice bag to the foot and arch area. Do not walk too much.

Severe Spasm: Attach an ice bag with elastic bandages to provide compression, and walk with crutches.

General Therapy

Add an arch support to the shoe to reduce further problems. See also "Foot Injuries," page 315.

ARM INJURIES

Ice therapy, with compression bandaging and elevation of the injured arm (if possible), is the usual initial treatment for arm injuries. Later, neutral arm baths will reduce congestion and quicken healing, and also lessen pain as well as formation of pus.

Arm area spasms should be treated with hot moist compresses.

BICEP STRAIN

In contact sports, the muscle under the biceps is greatly exposed and subject to repeated impact. This commonly leads to a contusion in the area.

Water Therapy

Apply an ice bag and pressure bandaging to quiet the bruise. Later soak the entire arm in apple cider vinegar and water, or apply diluted apple cider vinegar compresses.

General Therapy

Pad the bicep area after the first bruising, because the muscle under the bicep is very susceptible to additional bruising—especially with athletes—and repeated injury causes calcification.

"DEAD ARM"

The so-called "dead arm" is an acute and frightening experience that occurs in several sports, especially baseball. It is a result of a contusion to the arm that erupts suddenly in extreme radiating pain. "Dead arm" usually disappears in a few minutes, and rarely causes any permanent injury to the arm.

Water Therapy

Immediately apply several ice bags, or an ice pack made with a towel large enough to cover the entire arm.

General Therapy

Add padding to the arm. If the symptoms persist, see a physician.

ELBOW CUTS

A deeply penetrating laceration in the elbow often creates a secondary infection as well. This may result in a large swelling in the area.

Water Therapy

Wash the cut, and irrigate frequently in neutral-temperature elbow baths. Apply a local pressure bandage without drainage.

General Therapy

Immobilize the elbow in a sling for 8 to 10 days.

ELBOW STRAIN

Abnormal strain of the elbow (hyperextension) results in extreme tenderness and swelling.

Water Therapy

Immediately after the injury, apply ice to reduce the swelling.

General Therapy

After the initial ice therapy, place the elbow in a sling. These two therapies will reduce the swelling in 2 to 3 days.

Use an elbow cinch strapping to limit elbow extension. Gentle massage is also helpful. Use arnica lotion or Olbas oil to massage and reduce pain.

The elbow must be completely healed before the athlete returns to competition. Many trainers advise working out with a 20-pound bar to regain range of motion.

TENNIS ELBOW

Water Therapy

For a mild case, soak the elbow in a hot hand bath (105°F to 130°F). This has a general warming effect.

Reduce acute inflammation with a minimum 20-minute application of an ice bag or frozen bandage.

General Therapy

The elbow can often be snapped back into place in somewhat the same way a drawer is put back on its glides. Gently stretch the arm out, palm up, and put the elbow back in place.

Several herbal products, such as Olbas oil or ointment, arnica ointment, and wintergreen ointment, may be of help. A new product, Tennis Elbow Cream, is made from the anti-inflammation juice of the aloe vera plant (you may have such a plant in your house). The cream is said to penetrate the skin and soothe sore muscles and pulled ligaments. It is sold in some sporting goods stores and drugstores.

The "Don Joy Warm Up Sleeve" is a stretchable warmup sleeve that gives gentle pressure and some warmth to the area. It comes in three sizes and is also available for the knee and ankle.

FOREARM CONTUSION

This is a common injury in contact sports, where impact with football helmets or contact with the cleats on athletic shoes can cause painful multiple lacerations, bruises, or contusions.

Water Therapy

Immediately apply an ice bag to reduce internal bleeding. If there is no fracture, wrap the ice bag in an elastic pressure bandage and elevate the forearm with a sling. Afterward, use frequent neutral-temperature arm baths to speed healing and reduce the pain.

To further increase the circulation to the area, use these alternate hot and cold applications: hot and cold showers, hot and cold arm baths, hot and cold compresses.

FOREARM SPASM

This type of spasm frequently occurs to oarsmen.

Water Therapy

Apply hot moist compresses on the area of pain. Frequently plunge the entire arm into a neutral arm bath.

General Therapy

A week of self-paced stroking in a single shell will offset the pain and spasm.

BLISTERS

Water Therapy

As soon as you are aware of any localized friction burning on the foot or hands, place that part in cold water until the burning sensation stops. This technique, used by many athletic trainers, prevents blister formation. Trainers also use alum powder footbaths to harden the feet.

If a blister does form, massage the area with ice. Within a day this therapy reduces the excess fluid from the swelling and overcomes tenderness.

General Therapy

Wear white cotton socks under woolen socks. Apply calendula or a lanolin-based ointment on irritated spots. Use a moleskin to protect "hot" spots on the feet.

Shoes that fit properly are an absolute necessity, especially for sports activities. It also helps to break in shoes first.

BLISTER UNDER A CALLUS

Some athletes develop a blister under a callus. Be on the alert for these potentially painful blisters and prevent their formation with frequent Epsom salt soaks. Scrape the hardened skin with an emery board file. Do not use a knife.

BRUISES

Water Therapy

Routinely apply ice or a chilled substance to bruises. This controls the bleeding, inflammation, and swelling of the tissues and boosts the reabsorption of the congealed blood that makes up the bruise. Except for a bruised toenail or fingernail, which can be plunged into very hot water to relieve the swelling, never use heat on a bruise for the first 24 hours, as heat activates bleeding and spurs inflammation. Local heat only becomes advantageous 2 or 3 days after the bruise occurs.

ABRASION

An abrasion is a minor injury in which the superficial layers of the skin are removed. This can increase the vulnerability of the exposed skin layers to secondary infection.

Water Therapy

Wash the area with mild soap and warm water. Apply a local warm compress.

General Therapy

After washing, apply a healing lotion or ointment. Herb ointments such as calendula have outstanding healing powers. A slice of onion has remarkable healing powers and may be applied to the bruise. Sage tea compresses help with most bruises and expedite healing.

PALM BRUISE

The fleshy prominence of the palm near the little finger is prone to special bruises. Any such bruise should be carefully monitored, as it can sometimes develop into a small tumor (due to a new growth of blood vessels). Repeated striking, as in stick sports, can result in swelling, twinges of pain, and constriction of the blood to the area. This sometimes feels like needles and pins in the hand. Occasionally, this leads to an impaired sense of touch in the thumb and fingers, as in carpal tunnel syndrome.

Water Therapy

Take frequent alternate hot and cold arm baths, and alternate hot and cold compresses to increase circulation in the area. Direct alternate hot and cold jet shower streams to the area, and take alternate long hot and short cold showers.

General Therapy

Manual pressure therapy, physiotherapy, chiropractic, or Swedish massage can relieve the pressure due to weakness in the palm or wrist.

CONTUSION

A contusion is an injury with internal bleeding but no broken skin. The amount of the bleeding and swelling depend more on the location of the contusion than the extent of the injury. Soft tissues swell easily and must be attended to immediately.

Water Therapy

Apply ice immediately to stop the bleeding and control inflammation. Place a piece of fabric on the skin, and attach an ice-filled rubber bag with an elastic bandage to create a small amount of compression. Usually ice therapy is applied for 30 minutes, twice a day.

With superficial bruises, normal activity may be resumed fairly soon. Never use heat on a contusion for the first 24 to 48 hours, as heat restarts bleeding and provokes inflammation.

HEMATOMA

A hematoma is a tissue injury that swells and collects blood. The blood collection swells the tissues and creates a severe inflammation and local tenderness within the body.

Water Therapy

Place a molded rubber pad on the injury, apply an ice bag, and attach the bag with an elastic bandage to provide a slight compression. Also note specific instructions for each injury.

General Therapy

Continue ice therapy as directed for each injury. It is urgent to keep the blood collection at a minimum and reduce possible inflammation and swelling. Continue padding and compression for 7 to 10 days after the initial ice treatment.

A slice of onion may be applied under the ice. It will help to reduce the swelling as well as the pain.

SPRAIN

A sprain is a trauma to a joint that causes pain and disability depending on the degree of injury to the ligaments. In a severe sprain, ligaments may be torn completely. The ankle joint is often sprained, as is the wrist or knee joint. See specific instructions for ankle, wrist, and knee.

Water Therapy

Applying ice to the sprain or soaking the sprain in very cold water helps to alleviate pain and prevent further swelling. Cold-water compresses, with or without apple cider vinegar, witch hazel, or arnica lotion, may also be used. During rehabilitation, apply alternate hot and cold compresses and use whirlpool baths to increase circulation.

General Therapy

You can alternate apple cider vinegar, witch hazel, or arnica compresses, onion poultices, or onion and salt poultices, with the ice therapy. Onion slices may be applied directly to the sprain and attached with a bandage. The onion and salt application has excellent results. Combine equal amounts of grated onion with salt to make a paste and apply directly to injured area. Wrap with a bandage and overwrap with an elastic bandage. Keep the area moist with a plastic overwrap.

The onion poultices may be kept on overnight and repeated several nights in a row. This accelerates healing.

STRAIN

A strain is an injury resulting from excessive use of the body.

Water Therapy

Apply cold-water compresses and a firm dressing. Either elevate or immobilize the injured area.

General Therapy

In addition to immobilization, adhesive strapping may be necessary.

CLEAT BRUISES

Water Therapy

If there is no fracture, apply a wrapped ice bag to the bruise and attach with an elastic bandage. Elevate the area. This usually solves the problem within a day.

General Therapy

There will be extreme tenderness in the area. To prevent further impact, use rubber padding on the area for about 2 weeks. Apply a healing ointment such as calendula.

STRAWBERRY BRUISES

Water Therapy

A strawberry is a superficial abrasion of the skin that commonly occurs to sliding base runners. Immediately cleanse the strawberry with soap and warm water. This may smart. Calendula or chamomile tea may be used instead of soap and water for a more soothing effect.

General Therapy

Apply a nonsensitizing ointment such as calendula or comfrey to quickly heal the abrasion.

CALLUS

Water Therapy

Buildup of hardened tissue on the soles or the heels can interfere with normal or, especially, athletic activity. Prevent this buildup or soften the tissue by taking hot Epsom salt footbaths.

General Therapy

In addition to the footbaths, file the area with a special callus file. Do not hone the area with a razor blade. To maintain a soft and pliable foot, also rub a lanolin-based ointment into the callus and potential callus areas. Place a thin moleskin pad over the callus and attach with tape.

SWIMMER'S CALLUS

Water Therapy

Heal the cracked callus with herbal ointments such as calendula ointment. Then, harden the feet with frequent footbaths of cold to tepid water and alum, and also by treading in cold water. Increase foot circulation with alternate hot and cold showers.

General Therapy

Bleeding may occur in the edges of deep cracks along the edge of the foot because the water leeches out the natural oils of the body. Apply calendula ointment to heal the cracks.

CHEST STRAIN (PECTORAL STRAIN)

Water Therapy

A wild swing with a heavy object or too many pushups can create a chest strain. Besides feeling sore, there may also be swelling. This indicates some muscle fiber separation and bleeding.

If the area remains swollen for 24 to 48 hours, apply ice to the area of pain in 20-minute segments. Do this every 6 hours for 1 day.

General Therapy

Apply a sling to the arm on the side of the strain. If the strain occurs on both sides, suspend all activity that is even remotely strenuous. Symptoms tend to disappear within a few days unless there is swelling, in which case recovery may take about a week. Do not force movement. This injury must be allowed to heal naturally. Do not use painkillers. Because they mask the pain, they may cause a permanently torn pectoral muscle.

FLOATING RIBS

Water Therapy

Our ribs are constantly moving, but in young people the eleventh and twelfth ribs actually "float." A sharp impact to these two ribs results in swelling and pain, and causes difficulty in walking.

Ice therapy, used several times a day in 30-minute segments, will numb the initial pain and control swelling and possible internal bleeding.

General Therapy

This kind of injury usually occurs during athletic competition. The athlete must check with a physician and participate in a program of systematic and gradual exercises for a week before returning to competition.

SOLAR PLEXUS BLOW

Water Therapy

After the game, before going to sleep, relax in a long warm Epsom salt, mineral salt, table salt, or pine salt bath. End the bath with a cold friction massage.

Thereafter, direct alternate hot and cold shower streams from the midline under the breastbone to the navel to help circulation. Whenever possible, use cold-water therapies, especially cold-water treading, to reestablish body tone and energy.

General Treatment

An athlete who has been hit in the solar plexus develops an acute hunger for air and finds breathing difficult. Recovery from such a blow takes only a few minutes if the athlete is encouraged to relax and breathe rhythmically.

EYE INJURIES

BLACK EYES

Water Therapy

To slow internal bleeding and to reduce swelling and discoloration, apply anything cold to the area for only 10 minutes at a time each hour. The preferred application is an ice pack. If outdoors, use any available cold source including a can of soda or beer or a container of ice cream, or crushed ice in a plastic bag. Use a sweatband to attach the cold application. If something supercold is not available, apply a wet, cold compress. Repeat 10 minutes out of every hour, but temporarily withdraw the application if the person feels it is too cold.

General Therapy

After washing the area, apply a compress of witch hazel on the closed eye to reduce the puffiness, or use this ancient standby, a grated white potato encased in a handkerchief. Chamomile, thyme, parsley, and dandelion teas are also effective as individual compresses. To immediately increase the body's immune response, take additional doses of vitamin C and echinacea for at least two days following the incident.

FINGER INJURIES

CRUSHED FINGER

Water Therapy

Place the injured finger in cold water, and keep it in the water until the pain disappears. Add fresh cold water or ice water from time to time to keep the water cold. If preferred, a continuous cold compress may be applied.

SPORTS INJURIES

There are many ways to injure fingers during sports activities. Among the injuries are blisters, knuckle scrapes, knuckles bit or injured by human teeth, cuts, nail injuries, sprains, dislocations, and fractures.

Water Therapy

Apply an ice compress or miniature ice bag immediately to control bleeding and prevent swelling. Treat with ice for 30 minutes at a time. Apply over a finger splint.

Immediately soak any open finger wounds in rosemary tea. This promotes healing.

In between ice applications, apply arnica lotion or diluted arnica tincture to unbroken skin wounds. This reduces the pain. Olbas herbal oil or lotion also promotes healing.

Immerse the finger or arm in a neutral bath. These partial baths quicken healing.

See Resources for useful aids.

FOOT INJURIES

HEEL BRUISE

A heel bruise and the stone bruise of the metatarsal will be extremely tender for many months.

Water Therapy

Add arnica tincture to a neutral footbath and soak the foot for several hours each day. As often as possible, wrap a cold apple cider vinegar compress around the painful area of the foot.

Massage the area with herbal liniments or ointments, such as Olbas, eucalyptus, or wintergreen, which bring the blood to the surface.

SOLE OF THE FOOT INJURY

Common puncture wounds on the sole of the foot must always be checked by a doctor. Do not allow open wounds to become contaminated.

Water Therapy

Soak the foot daily in neutral salt water. Add tincture of St. John's wort or calendula tincture to water. Ledum tincture is also excellent. The wound should heal in 3 to 5 days.

FRACTURES

Fractures must be set by a professional.

Water Therapy

While waiting for the physician to arrive, or on the way to the hospital, fractures may be contained by applying ice bags. This controls internal bleeding.

Later during rehabilitation, you can improve blood circulation in arm and wrist fractures by frequently immersing the entire arm in hot water for

3 minutes, and then in cold water for 30 seconds. Repeat 3 times. Continue therapy as long as needed to restore normal mobility.

GENITAL INJURIES

BLOWS TO THE TESTICLES

Water Therapy

Blows to this area produce sudden ashen pallor, acute pain, and nausea.

Immediately apply ice packs. If bleeding continues, put the athlete to bed, give additional support to the testes, and apply ice packs intermittently. Sponge the area with strong rosemary tea. When the pain subsides, apply a hot compress. Alternate the hot compress with short cold spongings.

General Therapy

The testes should be examined by a physician within minutes of the injury if symptoms do not subside immediately. Even if they do subside, a physician or urologist should be consulted. The area may take months to reabsorb blood. After such an injury it is important to add additional cup support.

Fitted supporters are now mandatory in professional and intercollegiate sports, but not for very young players. Physicians dealing with sports injuries strongly advise the use of such supporters for all ages.

ROTATED TESTES

Water Therapy

After treatment by a urologist, cold sit baths and a genital compress will strengthen the area.

General Therapy

This rotation is rather rare, but it can occur in contact sports, particularly to men in their teens and twenties. The testes can sometimes be rotated into a 180° turn. Consult a urologist for any such testicular pain and swelling or rotation.

VULVA INJURIES

Water Therapy

When a fall astride the balance beam or parallel bar results in a contusion or laceration, immediately apply an ice pack for 20 minutes, and make sure to rest; both will minimize the bleeding.

Wash the area with calendula juice (*Succus calendula*) to stop the bleeding. This is a delicate aid and will help healing at the same time.

If there is no laceration, apply calendula ointment for the soothing and healing effect. If it is not available, pat on honey, for it will help reduce the feeling of irritation in the area and will heal. Honey is also useful for sores in the vulva.

General Therapy

Check any laceration with a physician.

GROIN STRAIN

Water Therapy

In sports, the complaint of a "tight" groin is so common that it is often ignored, and frequently leads to a disability that is even more difficult to cure and can last several weeks. This, in turn, may cause a season-long problem, or one that persists throughout all future athletic activity.

Immediately apply an ice bag to the area and hold it in place with an elastic bandage wound in a figure eight.

After the bleeding stops, use a program of alternate long hot and short cold showers to increase circulation to the area. Direct the shower to the area of pain. Occasional or nightly application of a double cold abdominal compress will reinvigorate and tone the area and have a general heating effect.

General Therapy

After the initial water therapy, the athlete must suspend play until the bleeding stops. During the healing process, use ointments and liniments that bring blood to the surface. These include wintergreen liniment, Olbas lotion or ointment, arnica lotion, mustard plaster, or cayenne pepper or ginger powder poultice.

Dr. Vincent Di Stephano, team physician for the Philadelphia Eagles, says he uses hot moist compresses as a secondary treatment if stiffness persists in the groin area.

Sitting in a cold whirlpool sit bath also helps.

An excellent preventive exercise that is used especially by skiers is to lift one foot onto a table or bathroom sink and stretch the groin area by leaning forward a half dozen times.

HAND INJURIES (SEE ALSO ARM INJURIES, FINGER INJURIES)

Water Therapy

Plunge the hand into containers of alternate hot and cold water. Plunge into hot water for 2 to 3 minutes and into cold water for 30 seconds. Repeat 6 times.

Neutral partial baths of the hand or arm will encourage the healing of any finger, hand, or arm injury.

KNUCKLES

A human tooth may occasionally create a minor wound on the knuckles during contact sports. Since this area can easily become infected, this injury should not be ignored.

Water Therapy

Cleanse the area with soap and water, and make sure the edges of the wound are clean. Do not close this wound. Keep checking the flexibility of the finger(s).

Soak the knuckle in diluted calendula lotion or calendula tincture to keep the wound clean and free of infection.

SORE WRIST

A sore wrist frequently indicates gripping a racket or bat too hard and/or not warming up sufficiently.

Water Therapy

Apply a hot moist heat compress on the wrist to relieve the spasm. Follow with a gentle cold friction massage on the wrist area.

Plunge the hand up to the elbow in neutral-temperature apple cider vinegar arm baths, and apply frequent apple cider vinegar compresses to the wrist.

Use whirlpool therapy to increase circulation.

JOCKSTRAP ITCH

Flareups of this ringworm infection occur more often in the summer, and may be brought on by tight clothing. This itch is sometimes complicated by secondary infections and methods of treatment.

Water Therapy

Observe the highest standards of personal cleanliness, as this fungus may persist indefinitely on the skin, or may repeatedly infect susceptible individuals.

For acute flareups, apply potassium permanganate compresses.

Use plenty of soap and water, germicide, and ointment. When bathing be sure to rinse away all soap and to carefully dry the area.

Wear cotton underwear. Boil it after each wearing.

KNEE INJURIES

Water Therapy

Ice is the initial treatment for a contusion, ligament sprain, laceration, muscle strain, tear, or fracture. Place a piece of clean cotton cloth over the injury and place an ice bag on top of the cloth. Attach with an elastic bandage. Elevate the knee. If you have a fracture, see a physician.

General Therapy

Check for hidden bleeding in all knee injuries. If you will be engaging in contact sport competition, attach a heavy protective pad of rubber or plastic under your uniform.

Massage torn ligaments with mixture of apple cider vinegar and iodized salt. Overcome stiffness and inflammation with neutral compresses dipped in apple cider vinegar and iodized salt. Apply the compress for 10 to 15 minutes.

CONTUSION

Water Therapy

Apply ice bags immediately, and repeat ice therapy at least twice a day (see above). Continue until the acute signs and symptoms of the bruise subside completely and a full range of motion is restored.

General Therapy

When the ice is removed, place a light foam rubber pad over the contusion area and secure it with an elastic bandage wrap. The objective is to render light compression to discourage hemorrhage and edema. Use a heavier rubber pad or plastic pad if you engage in contact sports activity.

KNEE SPRAINS

Water Therapy

Use the same therapy as for a contusion—ice, elastic adhesive strapping, felt splints, and elevation of the knee. Use crutches for ambulation.

Cold whirlpool therapy (65°F) helps mild and moderate sprains.

Apply apple cider vinegar and neutral to cold-water compresses, or vinegar and iodized salt packs, for 15 to 20 minutes.

General Therapy

Carefully examine the knee area for blood or lymph fluid that may escape into the knee tissues. According to Dr. Isao Hirata, Jr., of the University of South Carolina, any fluid escape beyond the second day may conceal cartilage damage.

After the initial ice treatment, Dr. Hirata puts his student athletes on a graduated jogging program. He feels that once motion is possible, proper control decreases the pain in the knee. After each workout, for the remainder of the season, Dr. Hirata applies a fresh supporting adhesive strapping to the knee. Between treatments, he suggests protecting the sprained area with additional foam rubber padding and elastic bandaging.

KNEE BURSITIS

Bursitis is an acute or chronic inflammation of a bursa. *Bursa,* a word we inherited from the Greeks, means a "wine skin," and is actually a sac or a saclike cavity filled with a viscous fluid and situated at places in the tissues at which friction would otherwise develop. The bursitis may be caused by a single or repeated trauma to the area.

Acute bursitis is characterized by pain, local swelling and tenderness, limited mobility of the affected area, and an escape of the fluid into the surrounding tissue. Due to scant blood supply in the area of joints, this leakage is rarely critical and is usually absorbed by the skin cells.

Water Therapy

Apply ice bags and elastic bandaging to relieve the swelling. Leave the ice bag on for 20 minutes. Repeat every 6 hours. The bleeding usually subsides in 1 or 2 days, and another 2 days is needed for the swelling to reduce. Retain the elastic bandaging, and apply additional padding to the knee area in future athletic activities.

Acute cases of bursitis respond to ice massage. Rotate the ice on the skin of the knee until the area responds with pain. Alternate the ice massage with a warm palming of the same area. Once the area warms up, massage with ice again. Repeat this sequence 3 or 4 times.

Just before bedtime, follow the ice massage with 1 or 2 applications of an ice bandage (frozen washcloth). The washcloths will warm up as you use them. Afterward, dry the knee and wrap it in a wool or flannel cloth in order to keep the area warm. Wear pajamas to bed to retain the warmth.

General Therapy

After injury to the area or swelling from an injury, temporarily cease all athletic activity. The usual recovery period is 1 to 2 weeks, but the condition may become chronic if you resume activity too soon.

BEHIND THE KNEECAP (FAT PAD)

The area behind the kneecap is often bruised in normal sports activities, particularly in the running, jumping, and kicking sports. This pinching of the pad may be visible only as a minor bruise, but stress creates repeated squeezing of the area that may lead to additional bleeding and leaking of fluid into the kneecap area.

Water Therapy

An ice bag, ice bandage, or ice massage will help to control bleeding and check swelling.

KNEE CUTS

Cuts, particularly deep lacerations, are quite painful in the knee area. Because of the dead space in the knee (and the elbow), the area is more susceptible to secondary infection.

Water Therapy

Cleanse and irrigate the cut. Apply a local pressure dressing without drainage.

General Therapy

Cuts respond well to the following herbal preparations: calendula lotion, calendula tincture (diluted), or the pure juice of the pot marigold (*Succus calendula*). Diluted St. John's wort (*Hypericum perforatum*) helps in the healing of deep cuts; diluted tincture of ledum helps with puncture wounds.

KNEE DISLOCATION

Immediate replacement of the knee decreases the pain, swelling, and spasm in the entire area. See a physician and have an X ray taken to check for internal injury.

Water Therapy

Apply an ice bag, pressure bandage, and felt splint for 30 minutes at a time until pain, swelling, and spasm are decreased.

Do not apply any weight to the knee joint. Use crutches for walking.

There is considerable controversy among orthopedists on the necessity and usefulness of knee operations to correct dislocation. Some physicians note that the long-term results of knee operations are negligible.

KNEE JOINT INFLAMMATION

Water Therapy

Edgar Cayce advises applying packs made of apple cider vinegar and iodized salt. Leave packs on for 4 to 5 hours.

SNAPPING EXTENSION OF THE KNEE

A snapping extension of the knee should be checked by a physician. Often when the knee is flexed, the physician discovers that the muscle that is largely affected is the large muscle of the back of the calf.

Water Therapy

Apply an ice bag, or massage with an ice cube for 10 to 15 minutes every few hours.

Most athletes are back in action in less than a week and have no additional knee damage.

MUSCLES

CRAMPS

Water Therapy

Hand Cramps: Immerse hands in hot hand baths for cramps due to tennis, typing, piano playing, writing, ham radio work, potting, painting, gardening, or factory work.

Leg Cramps: Apply hot moist compresses on the legs to relieve pain and increase local circulation. Or simultaneously immerse the feet up to the knees in a hot footbath and apply a hot moist compress to the inner thighs and knees.

General Therapy

Most chronic muscle cramps are due to the inability of the body to assimilate certain needed materials, or from a mineral or vitamin deficiency, such as a hydrochloric acid deficiency.

Having enough vitamin E may help alleviate leg cramps. Magnesium, potassium, and the vitamins B_6, C, and D are also important in preventing leg cramps. Add a whole B supplement or brewer's yeast tea made from licorice and tea made from ginseng powder or extract to the diet. These are said to increase natural hormones in the body, and may help with endocrine imbalance.

CALF CRAMPS

Water Therapy

Many people have painful nighttime cramps. Hot whirlpool baths will relieve the problem temporarily. However, any other local heat applications or ice may bring on additional spasms. It greatly helps to knead any knots before, during, and after the whirlpool baths.

When the cramps are due mainly to athletic or dance activity, it may be because the body has been depleted of water and salt. Add a small amount of salt to your drinking water, or take several salt tablets before performances, practice, or competition. Salt must be flushed down with lots of water.

Also drink lots of water before, during, and after all athletic or dance activities.

General Therapy

Increase your calcium and vitamin C intake. Eat foods high in potassium.

ATROPHIED MUSCLES

Water Therapy

Apply alternate hot and cold compresses; direct alternate hot and cold showers to the atrophied muscles; or immerse the atrophied area in alternate hot and cold partial baths.

STIFF MUSCLES

Water Therapy

Hot baths, especially when they contain a cup or two of Epsom salts, are a great defense against stiff muscles. The effect of such a bath is magnified when the following herbal ointments are massaged on the stiff areas prior to and after the bath: Tiger Balm, Olbas ointment, wintergreen oil, homeopathic arnica. Always take Epsom salt baths at night before retiring, as these baths are not only relaxing and detoxifying, but tend to temporarily deplete one's energy and thus encourage sleepiness.

Stiff, aching muscles are an ancient problem. This is an old fisherman's liniment: Combine 1 cup of hot apple cider vinegar, 1/2 teaspoon of cayenne pepper, 6 drops of pine oil, and 1 tablespoon of dried seaweed.

SWOLLEN MUSCLES

Apply cold compresses to swellings.

TORN OR STRAINED MUSCLES

Apply alternate hot and cold compresses to the area of the pain to increase circulation and oxygen to the area.

NECK TENSION

Water Therapy

Many of us carry our tension in our shoulders and neck. One way to decompress the area is to take a long, leisurely, full hot bath with the water high enough to reach the neck. Place a steamy-hot towel across the shoulder blades and neck area and a cold compress on the forehead, and relax! Pine oil extract, drops of valerian tincture, or drops of melissa tea may be added to the bath. If your neck is extremely stiff or tense, you can intensify the relief from the hot water by patting some homeopathic arnica ointment or Tiger Balm ointment on the neck and shoulders just before getting into the bath.

If there is no time for a leisurely bath, steep your feet in moderately hot bathwater for 5 to 10 minutes. This will help to divert the congestion from the neck area to the lower extremities.

WATER'S EFFECTS ON MUSCLES

Short cold water application	Increases muscle ability and range
Long cold application	Lessens muscle capability and response
Short hot application	Reduces muscle fatigue
Long hot application	Lessens muscle ability and response

SHIN INJURIES

BARKED SHIN

Water Therapy

Apply ice immediately to the skin, use elastic bandaging to hold the ice, and elevate the lower leg. Do this for 30 minutes every few hours for 24 to 48 hours, to prevent secondary phlebitis.

If the area does become inflamed, it will be necessary to go to bed. Then apply hot moist compresses and elevate the lower leg. This will probably clear the inflammation within a week.

General Therapy

Even minor injuries to this area of the lower leg can be painful. Lack of attention to this injury, and forcing athletic activity too soon afterward, can lead to a very serious condition called a thrombus. A thrombus is a collection of blood trapped with cells, which can cause an obstruction in blood circulation.

When running activities are resumed, use protective padding.

SHIN SPLINTS

Water Therapy

There is no specific water treatment for this condition, but treading in cold water will strengthen the feet and the entire body.

General Therapy

Pain in the area below the knee has been termed shin splints in the general press. It is a chronic problem, but many years ago, Yale trainer O. W. Dayton observed that the reason for this chronic pain was foot rotation. "Athletes with shin splints always walk duck-footed!" Dayton observed.

Over the course of many years, Dayton discovered a painless method of correcting the problem. Each day, Dayton strapped the ankles of athletes who rotated their feet, and he reversed the rotation. By taping the foot so that it would be inverted, and by instituting workouts in pigeon-toed steps, most of the Yale athletes overcame the problem within a month.

Today, such rotations are usually brought to the attention of a parent by a pediatrician. When a child is 13 months old or so, an orthopedist can change his or her walk so that the stride will be normal.

SHOULDER INJURIES

Water Therapy

Several home measures will help to overcome general injury pain in the shoulder area. Initially, apply an ice bag for 20 minutes every several hours for 24 hours after the impact. Also use an arm sling for 24 hours.

Follow the ice and sling treatment with moist heat applications to the injured area. Hot showers are best, but frequent hot moist compresses are also beneficial.

After several days, direct alternate long hot showers and brief cold showers to the injury. This will increase circulation and speed healing.

Olbas lotion, arnica lotion, or wintergreen liniment will relieve some pain.

General Treatment

Severe impact during contact sports can cause painful internal bruises in the shoulder area with consequent tenderness and swelling. For this reason, it is vital to lessen potential impact with shoulder pads that fit well and are close to the body and neck. The jersey must also fit tightly over the shoulder pads to prevent the pads from sliding.

DELTOID STRAIN

Water Therapy

The back and front deltoid strains are treated in the same way. Apply ice to the area of the pain. Then strap the shoulder cap from the top of the shoulder to the upper arm with several narrow adhesive strips. Over these, place additional strips that run in the direction of the chest to the back, or strips that run in armband style. Elevate the injury with a sling. Reapply ice periodically for 24 hours.

After a day or two—depending on the severity of the injury—switch to hot shower therapy. Continue for several days. In order to increase the elasticity of the tissues and aid mobility, Dr. Vincent Di Stephano, orthopedic specialist and team physician for the Philadelphia Eagles, prefers to use heat, especially moist heat, at this point prior to motion exercises. He then uses whirlpool therapy or hot showers directed to the injured part.

DELTOID BURSITIS

Water Therapy

Apply ice bags and elastic bandaging to relieve the swelling. If there is internal bleeding, it takes 1 or 2 days to subside, and about 2 more days for the swelling to be reduced.

Just as with knee bursitis, acute cases respond to ice massage. Rotate the ice on the painful area until you are uncomfortable, and alternate the ice massage with warm palming of the muscle. Repeat several times.

Frozen or ice bandages are useful at this time. Apply these bandages in a series of two, prior to bedtime. Dry the area well, and attach a flannel cloth or wear a flannel shirt to keep the muscle warm.

General Therapy

Until pain and tenderness have subsided, keep your arm rested in a sling (except during a graduated program of exercises).

SHOULDER DISLOCATION

Water Therapy

No water therapy will prevent or cure this problem, but frequent alternate long hot showers and brief cold showers will increase the tone and circulation of the shoulder area.

General Therapy

Dislocation is quite frequent in contact sports because of the shallowness of the shoulder area. The best remedy is for an expert to immediately replace the bone. Relief can be instantaneous if the expert's foot-in-the-armpit traction is utilized.

After the first dislocation, the shoulder can have a tendency to slip out again. Even simple activities, such as shampooing, can push out the round knob at the upper end of the arm bone.

FROZEN SHOULDER

Water Therapy

To reduce the pain and inflammation on the shoulder, apply an ice pack for 20 minutes at a time. Repeat during the first 2 days as often as possible. After 48 hours, heat can be used.

Alleviate the pain with alternate long bursts of hot and brief barrages of cold showers. Always end with a cold application.

General Therapy

Alleviate pain, trauma, and inflammation by taking 1 to 3 pills of homeopathic arnica 6x under the tongue. Also apply homeopathic arnica ointment to the stiff shoulder. Other effective topical ointments are Olbas oil, Tiger Balm, and wintergreen liniment.

LOOSE SHOULDERS

Water Therapy

Alternate long hot showers and brief cold showers to the shoulder area will increase the total muscle tone and vitality. Hot moist compresses will relieve pain.

General Therapy

A loose shoulder can develop from repeated impact during wrestling or football.

SHOULDER SEPARATION (POINTER)

Water Therapy

Apply an ice bag for 30 minutes several times a day. Strap the shoulder cap and elevate the arm in a sling for several days.

After 2 days, direct hot showers to the area of injury. Whirlpool therapy is also used by William E. "Pinky" Newell of Purdue University.

A gradual exercise program should be started at this time and continued until there is a full range of movement in the shoulder.

The athlete may return to competition in about 6 days after the initial water treatments. Add additional protective padding to the shoulder area.

General Therapy

Minor separations are relieved by water therapy and a sling. Major separations of a few millimeters or more must be rigidly strapped.

GENERAL RELAXATION

Water Therapy

Take warm baths. Sit deep in the bath with the water up to your neck. Place a light hand towel on the shoulders to reinforce the water action. Rotate each shoulder forward and back. Do slow neck rolls to relax the neck.

If the neck is very tense, apply a warm compress around the neck while in the bath. A hydrocallator hot neck pack can be used. These silica-gel aids retain heat (or cold). They are available in most drugstores.

GENERAL SHOULDER PAIN

Water Therapy

Shoulder pain may mean there is an imbalance in the gall bladder or liver. To reach the liver area and increase its activity, direct a short cold shower to the lower right chest and abdomen, and directly over the liver area.

To relax the muscles of the bile duct and gall bladder, apply a large hot moist compress or a hot pack to the trunk of the body. This may relieve the pain if it is due to a spasm of these muscles.

An alternate long hot and short cold (Scots) shower directed from the midline of the ribs to the midline of the abdomen relieves shoulder and intercostal pain.

The following herbal poultices are also useful: hot moistened flaxseed, cooked marshmallow root, cooked hot comfrey root, moistened comfrey leaves, and gingerroot tea. Place any of these in a handkerchief, light kitchen towel, or cloth, and apply to the area of pain.

SPRAIN AND SWELLING

Water Therapy

Immediately apply an ice pack to the sprain for 20 minutes an hour during the first 24 hours. This reduces recovery time as well as potential inflammation. Practice RICE: Rest, Icing, Compression, and Elevation. Compression means either light bandaging or an elastic bandage such as sold by Ace.

After the first 24 hours—sometimes 48 hours—it is possible to apply heat. For sprains, it is best to employ alternate long hot and brief cold shower applications to the area of the sprain or swelling.

To reduce the swelling and inflammation apply cloths soaked in witch hazel extract or apple cider vinegar compresses to the area of the sprain.

For severe limb swelling soak the foot or hand in Burrow's solution (obtained in drugstores.)

Bromelain, the enzyme in fresh pineapple, blocks the internal compounds that produce additional inflammation and swelling in the body. Drink lots of pineapple juice, eat fresh pineapple, or take bromelain capsules.

Reduce swelling by applying cabbage leaves to the area. Discard the first outer leaves because they usually have large, heavy veins. Dip a cabbage leaf in extremely hot water to further diminish the cabbage's vein, and fasten it around the swollen area.

General Therapy

Supplementation with coenzyme Q10 may help protect athletes against exercise-induced muscle injury. Use citrus bioflavonoid supplements to reduce the recovery time of swelling due to sports injuries. Heat a leaf of an aloe plant and apply to any swollen area to reduce swelling. The swelling from arthritis can be lessened with large doses of ginger throughout the day. It may be eaten in food or taken as a capsule.

STITCH

A stitch is an acute pain, usually on the right side. It is disabling because it is virtually impossible to breathe properly for several minutes during this kind of attack.

One of the most effective ways of regaining mobility is to lie down with upraised arms and rest for 10 to 15 minutes. If it occurs during a sports activity, the athlete can then return to competition. Such attacks rarely return for at least a few weeks, if at all.

Water Therapy

Apply a single cold abdominal compress to tone the abdominal organs and overcome gas in the colon or stomach. Direct alternate hot and cold showers to the area from the midline under the breastbone to the navel. Tone up the heart area with occasional cold compresses. Tread in cold water to increase circulation throughout the system and to tone the entire body.

General Therapy

The cause of a stitch is not actually known, but several theories speculate on these possible causes: gas in the colon, gas in the stomach, or a brief swelling of the liver from a temporary heart insufficiency.

TENDINITIS

Tendinitis, an inflammation of a tendon and its lining, is to be treated as a sprain by using rest, icing, compression, and elevation (RICE).

Water Therapy

Repeated applications of a frozen bandage draws instant blood to the area. This allows the area to heat up from within to initiate a unique healing process. As each cloth heats up, discard it and apply fresh cloths. This series of iced bandages can stand alone as a treatment, or you may also do the following:

1. Gently massage adjacent areas along the length of the tendon.
2. After the massage apply an ice pack for 10 minutes.

Witch hazel extract is one of the best antiswelling herbs in our pharmacopoeia. Apply "neat" from the bottle to reduce heat and swelling on the body.

Heated paraffin dips are excellent for tendinitis as well as foot injuries and arthritic pains. Such paraffin treatments are frequently available at physiotherapist and massage offices or a paraffin wax machine may be obtained via mail-order sources. (See Resources.)

General Therapy

Ferrum phos. is the homeopathic cell salt used in the initial stage of any inflammation. During the acute stage take 5 tablets of ferrum phos. 6x every half-hour to an hour. When the swelling, pain, and hardness of the tendinitis diminishes, lengthen the intervals between the doses. Homeopathic arnica tablets are an excellent remedy to counteract trauma and pain.

The dose of arnica 6x may be repeated up to 5 times a day. Arnica also can be purchased in ointment form. Other topical antipain ointments are Tiger Balm, aloe, or wintergreen lotion, but these should not be used at the same time as any homeopathic remedy. During an acute stage of tendinitis, bromelain or turmeric capsules can also be used topically as poultices. Mix the contents of one or two capsules with a small amount of water to make a paste. Place the paste on a soft cotton cloth or gauze and apply damp on the area of pain. Such capsules may also be taken internally to further reduce inflammation.

Nutritional aids to counter tendinitis include daily use of anti-inflammatory black currant seed or borage oil capsules as well as antioxidants such as vitamin C, vitamin E, and selenium to quench newly loosed free radicals. Vitamin C helps to repair damage and restore collagen and should be used along with vitamin E, and such flavonoids as quercetin and the citrus bioflavonoids, which shorten injury-recovery time. In addition, use zinc to encourage tissue repair. The herb St. John's wort is an ancient wound aid that came into prominence during the Crusades. Clinical studies show it has strong anti-inflammatory action when taken internally, one capsule a day.

THIGH INJURIES

CHARLEY HORSE FROM CONTUSION

Heavy impact in the area of the thigh can create massive internal bleeding that can then lead to an almost crippling charley horse.

The player should be pulled from the game immediately. Preventing aggravation of the injury is of primary concern.

Water Therapy

Immediately apply ice packs and elastic bandaging, and elevate the thigh. Two hours later, evaluate the situation. If the thigh is slightly better, continue the treatment for another 48 hours. However, if the pain and swelling stay at the same level, the case is serious. With a moderate charley horse injury, an athlete may walk on crutches; if it is a severe injury, he or she must be immobilized.

Continue the ice therapy for 30 to 60 minutes twice a day until the acute signs are gone. Between each ice application, apply a foam rubber pad over the bruised area and attach it with an elastic bandage. This should provide a light tension pressure. Remove the foam rubber when the ice bag is applied.

Under no circumstances apply heat in any form to this bruise. A warm shower is permitted if the ice bag is wrapped over the thigh bruise.

Do not use ice massage on this bruise.

General Therapy

This is a very common injury. Dr. A. Kalenak of Pennsylvania State University notes in *The Physician and Sports Medicine* that this injury is often ignored, especially on the community, high school, and junior college levels where athletes are often told to "run it out," or "suck it up"—"This inappropriate treatment results in prolonged recovery, and even permanent disability from loss of muscle strength and flexibility."

One way to avoid a charley horse in football is to insist on a properly fitted pants shell in which the protective padding provided for the thigh stays in place.

Once the bleeding stops, Dr. Isao Hirata, Jr., of South Carolina University suggests stretching exercises, heel to buttock exercises, and a gradual walking program working into jogging and running.

If a massive charley horse occurs, when the bleeding stops, apply hot moist compresses for a week and stay off your feet.

HAMSTRING INJURY

Water Therapy

Every 2 hours, apply an ice bag and bandage with plastic so that there is some compression. Leave the ice bag on for 30 minutes. If the muscle goes into a spasm, it may indicate a muscle pull or internal bleeding.

General Therapy

Walk normally after the bleeding stops. Gradually do high knee exercises and jogging. If the bleeding is heavy, delay activity for about 2 weeks.

MIDDLE THIGH

Water Therapy

Apply an ice bag for 20 minutes every few hours.

General Therapy

Place padding in the area of injury and resume activity in about 5 days. Middle thigh (adductor) muscle injury is not too serious.

TOE INJURIES

SPRAIN OF THE BIG TOE

Water Therapy

A big toe sprain responds superficially to an ice bag, elastic bandaging, and elevation of the toe. Soak the entire foot in ice cold apple cider vinegar, or apply apple cider vinegar compresses to reduce the feeling of pain and strain.

General Therapy

This may look like a small injury, but it can keep an athlete on the sidelines for up to 2 weeks. As this is the weight-bearing toe, it must be healed before any athletic activity can resume.

To somewhat reduce the pain, apply arnica lotion to the toe.

SPRAINS OF OTHER TOES

Water Therapy

Apply ice as soon as possible for 30 minutes at a time, several times during the day.

General Therapy

All the toes (except the big toe) can be strapped to any other healthy toe, and the athlete can go back into action immediately.

STIFF BIG TOE

Water Therapy

Soak the foot in apple cider vinegar or hayflower water. If the stiffness is a result of some infection, take hayflower baths several times a week. Use frequent cold water friction massage on the entire body.

General Therapy

A chronic stiff big toe can result from an injury or athletic shoes that are too tight, or may indicate an infection in the teeth or tonsils or elsewhere in the body.

Often physicians encase the foot in a plaster cast for 6 weeks, and provide a bar under the sole of the shoe for a few months. The bar allows rocking motion of the foot and this helps the tender joint of the toe.

resources

THERAPY PRODUCTS USING WATER

Steam Inhaler: Bernhard Steam Inhaler. Bronson Pharmaceuticals, 4426 Rinetti Lane, PO Box 628, La Canada, CA 91012-0628; 1-800-732-3323. The inhaler is only 7½ inches tall, weighs 16 ounces, converts to local voltage anywhere, uses tap water; provides drugless relief for congestions, colds, or sinus, throat, and allergy conditions.

Footbath/Face Sauna: Attitudes, 1-800-525-2468. Portable footbath includes reflex massage pad, heat, and whirlpool bubbles; face sauna has directed steam for sinus relief, aromatherapy, and skin cleansing.

Sitz Bath: Duro-Med, Hackensack, NJ: for local distributor, call 1-800-525-2468. Half-bath for lower extremities.

Humidifier: Portable 4- to 6-gallon model. Hammacher Schlemmer, 147 East 57th Street, New York, NY 10022; 1-800-283-9400. Claims to eliminate up to 97 percent of bacteria found in most mist; also to remove dust, smoke, and irritants in air. Demineralizer eliminates white dust residue.

Hot Water Bottle: Hard-to-find British flannel-clad hot water bottle. Vermont Country Store, PO Box 1108, Route 7, North Manchester Center, VT 05255; (802) 362-4647. Use instead of electric heating pad.

HOME SAUNAS, HOT TUBS, WHIRLPOOLS, STEAM BATHS

Built-In Sauna Rooms, Steam Rooms, Accessories: Thermasol, 1-800-631-1601 (eastern), 1-800-776-1711 (western).

Hot Tubs, Steam Rooms, Saunas, Whirlpools: Baths and Spas International, 1-800-875-2600.

Portable Whirlpools: Jacuzzi, 1-800-288-4002.

BATH PRODUCTS

Detoxifying: Hayflower Bath Extract. Biokosma, Switzerland; available at better health stores and from Caswell-Massey (oldest pharmacy in the U.S.); call 1-800-326-0500 for catalog. Extract of alpine flowers, horse chestnut, and juniper, for use in bath or compresses.

Mustard Bath: Dr. Singha's Mustard Bath. Natural Therapeutics Centre, 2500 Side Cove, Austin, TX 78704; (512) 444-2862. Formulated by Dr. Shyam Singha, a London acupuncturist and naturopath, this is made of powder from English mustard seeds and essential oils of eucalyptus, rosemary, wintergreen, and thyme; stimulates circulation and relieves aches and pains of cold; best used as a footbath to forestall a cold.

Varied Bath Products: The Body Shop; call 1-800-541-2535 for catalog. This British-based firm specializes in products made with natural ingredients such as herbal bath oils, massage oils, Body Buddy rubber mitt, and exfoliating cactus brushes and mitts.

HERBAL PRODUCTS

Aloe Products: Aloe Flex Products, 1-800-231-0839. This Texas company grows its own aloe for topical use for tennis elbow, carpal tunnel syndrome, and burns (including radiation burns).

Arnica Tablets: Health food stores and drugstores carrying homeopathic products; The Vitamin Shoppe; call 1-800-223-1216 for catalog of homeopathic items. For body trauma, aches, pains, postsurgical problems, and for use before dental surgery.

Calendula Ointment: Available at health food stores or from Weleda; call 1-800-241-1030 for catalog. This healing salve is made from marigolds. Weleda also makes a variety of all-natural body care products from their own gardens, where they practice companion planting and other natural methods to eliminate pests. Products include chamomile extract, arnica massage oil, body lotions, baby care products, and mouth products.

Castor Oil: Palma Christi Castor Oil. The Heritage Store, PO Box 44-U, Virginia Beach, VA 23458-0444. For effective healing compresses and packs.

Melisana: M.C.M. Klosterfrau, D 5000 Cologne 1, Germany. A remarkable German carminative (antigas treatment) made from an ancient convent recipe. A few drops in a glass of water are used for gastric relief; can also be used topically for muscle soreness.

Olbas Massage Oil, Analgesic Oil, Ointment, and Lotion: Available at health food stores or call Penn Herb Co., Ltd., Philadelphia, PA, 1-800-523-9771 for catalog.

Slippery Elm Lozenges: Available at health food stores or write to Henry Thayer Company, PO Box 56, Westport, CT 06881-0056, (203) 226-0940, www.thayers.com. These have been comforting irritated throats for a century and a half.

Swedish Bitters: Available at health food stores or GNC or call Nature Works, Inc., at 1-800-226-6227, www.natureworks.com. An herbal tonic and restorative with 10 herbs plus aloe (a laxative when taken internally).

Tiger Balm: Available at health food stores and drugstores. An Asian herbal analgesic ointment, available in white and red formulations; the red is stronger but may stain clothes. Alternate with arnica ointment for muscle and other aches; a whiff of Tiger Balm may avert a sinus attack.

Zostrix: In pharmacy section of drugstores, but it's a nonprescription item. This topical analgesic's active ingredient is capsaicin (cayenne pepper); intended for relief of arthritis pain and neuralgias such as shingles (herpes zoster) or diabetic neuropathy. One of the few things besides cool compresses, Aveeno, and witch hazel compresses that can make life bearable during a shingles attack.

ALLERGY AIDS

Negative Ion Generator: The Sharper Image, 1-800-344-5555.

Enviracaire Air Filtering System: Walnut Acres, Penns Creek, PA 17862, 1-800-283-9400. Said to remove tobacco smoke, bacteria, pollen, dust, chemical fumes, pet hair, lint, and other pollutants.

Humidifier: Hammacher Schlemmer; see listing under "Therapy Products Using Water," on page 339.

BABY PRODUCTS

All these are available from One Step Ahead, PO Box 517, Lake Bluff, IL 60044; for questions and catalog, call 1-800-950-2120, weekdays 8 A.M.–11 P.M. Central Time; for orders, call 1-800-274-8440; fax (708) 615-2162.

Newborn Bathing: Baby Bather. This unique item is for that crucial time up to five months, when young parents are so tense. I remember taking the easy way and bathing my beloved in a small portable plastic "tub" in the kitchen sink. Now someone has invented a soft-as-air contour cushion that not only frees your hands but cradles the baby.

Six Months to Two Years: Baby Mooring Seat. No more slippery babies in the tub. Here is a collapsible, fitted seat that attaches to the tub, with easy straps for the baby. Your hands are miraculously free to make the child happy and comfortable.

Parent Knee Saver: Bathe'r Save'r. Older parents would have killed for this padded knee mat! Kneeling was never such fun.

Double Duty: Apron/Towel Hugger. Big enough for Mom or Dad, and when the bath ends you can hug the baby dry.

SINUS AIDS

Neti Pot: For nasal irrigation. Available through the Himalayan Institute, 1-800-822-4547.

Grossan Nasal Irrigator: Available through pharmacies or through Hydromed Inc., (310) 372-8801.

TheraSteam Personal Inhaler KZ-0100: Opens up obstructed sinuses by concentrating vapor to the nose. Available at InteliHealth Healthy Home Catalog, 1-800-988-1127.

Sinus Mask with Heat/Cold, SW-0100: Available at InteliHealth Healthy Home Catalog, 1-800-988-1127.

ASTHMA AIDS

Bionaire Clear Mist: A tabletop humidifier. Call 1-800-253-2764 (U.S.) or 1-800-561-6478 (Canada) for local stores.

Kenmore Warm Mist: Tabletop humidifier, available at most Sears stores.

Bernhard Steam Inhaler: Available at 1-800-544-6425.

Eucalyptus Oil: To buy eucalyptus oil for steam inhalers, try health food stores or V-Vax products, (312) 276-1747.

AIR PURIFIERS

Negative Ion Generators: Available through Air Tech International, (303) 530-3934, and some hardware and department stores.

HEPA Air Cleaners: Available in many hardware and department stores. Check your local Yellow Pages.

Bionaire F-150: A combination air purifier/ion generator. Call 1-800-253-2764 (U.S.) and 1-800-561-6478 (Canada) for local stores.

Furnace Filter: "The Magnet" (Magnet High Efficiency Allergy Relief Filter), available at hardware stores and Sears, or call 1-800-288-8955.

Test Kit for Indoor Allergens (Dust Mite, Mold, Roach, Cat): Available at Healthy Habitats, (303) 671-9653.

Personal Air Purifier, T213314: Wear around your neck; wonderful for long flights. Brookstone mail-order catalog, 1-800-926-7000.

NONTOXIC CLEANERS

Dupont Wizard Dustcloth: Available at Healthy Habitats, (303) 671-9653.

Dupont Hysurf Vacuum Cleaner Bags: Available at Healthy Habitats, (303) 671-9653.

MOTION SICKNESS

Acupressure Wristbands: Available from Travel Accessories, (216) 248-8432.

COLD/HOT PACK

Aromapac Neck Wraps, Back Cushions, and Foot Pillows: Packs filled with herbs such as eucalyptus and cloves. Can be heated or cooled. Call Living Arts Catalog, 1-800-254-8464, www.livingarts.com.

Shoulder Wraps, Neck Wraps, Foot and Arm Wraps, Hot/Cold, Velcro Closures: Intelihealth, 1000 Intelihealth Plaza, Ridgely, MD 21685, 1-800-988-1127, www.intelihealth.com.

WATER FOOT MASSAGE

Jet Action Whirlpool Foot Massager, EB-0100: Available at Intelihealth Healthy Home, 1-800-988-1127.

SAUNA

AromaSpa Steam Capsule: For one or two; available at Intelihealth Healthy Home, 1-800-988-1127.

BATHTUB WHIRLPOOL

Home Whirlpool Spa, HY-0200: Available at Intelihealth Healthy Home, 1-800-988-1127.

PARAFFIN HEAT THERAPY

Therabath Paraffin Heat Therapy System: Available at Intelihealth Healthy Home, 1-800-988-1127.

SUPPORT GROUPS FOR CHRONIC FATIGUE SYNDROME

Meeting and talking with someone who has the same symptoms and problems can often be a turnaround for a patient with CFS. CFS Survival Association (PO Box 1889, Davis, CA 95617) will provide names of other patients, resources, and referrals to support groups.

CFIDS Association of America (Chronic Fatigue Immune Dysfunction), PO Box 220398, Charlotte, NC 28222, 1-800-44-CFIDS, www.cfids.org. The organization publishes a quarterly magazine, *The CFIDS Chronicle,* with current research and access to information.

index

A

abdominal area, 25
    cold double compress or pack for,
      58–59
    showering, 133
abrasions, 307
abscess, 225
    general therapy, 158
    water therapy, 157–58
Achilles tendon, 300
acid drinks, 39
acidophilus, 227
acne
    general therapy, 159
    water therapy, 158–59
Airola, Paavo, 265
Air Power (Enzymatic Therapy), 244
air purifiers, 205
alcohol drinking, and drinking
      water, 38
Algemarin, 101, 103
    effects in bathwater, 100

allergies
    to foods, 253
    hay fever, 204–5
    inflammatory bowel disease and,
      226–27
    to local water, 36
alternate applications of heat and cold
    footbath, 90–91
    hand bath, 97
    legbath, 91–92
    shallow bath, 78
    showers, 131–32
    therapeutic uses, 28, 32
    types of, 32
aluminum
    Alzheimer's disease and, 11
    leaching of, 11
Alzheimer's disease, 11
anal area, 32, 61–62, 225, 231
    bidet for, 135
anesthetic, water as, 22
    techniques, 22

angina, 209–10
ankle injuries, water therapy for, 300–2
    arch spasm, 302
    bone bruise, 302
    forefoot, 301
    sprain, 300
    weak ankles, 300
ankle splash, cold-water, 147
antacids, 39
antibiotics, overuse of, 6
antiseptic, water as, 21
antispasmodic, water as, 22
    techniques, 22
A'o, Lono Kahuna Kupua, 13
apple cider vinegar, 117, 163, 181
    baths, 20, 101
    compresses, 48, 52
    effects in bathwater, 100
    hair rinse, 116
aquifers, 11
arm and footbath, simultaneous, 146
arm injuries, therapy for, 302–6
    bicep strain, 303
    "dead arm," 303
    elbow cuts, 303–4
    elbow strain, 304
    forearm contusion, 305
    forearm spasm, 305–6
    tennis elbow, 304–5
arnica, 51
    compresses, 48
arteries, 30
arthritis
    clay poultice for pain, 154
    dehydration and, 16
    drinking water and, 37
    water therapy, 159–61
ascorbic acid bath, 112–13
aspirin, 11
asthma
    dehydration and, 16
    general therapy, 164
    water therapy, 162–63
athletes
    exercise recovery, 300

finger injuries, 314
fluid intake, 38–39
salt intake, 38–39, 324
shin injuries, 326–27
shoulder injuries, 327–31
stitch in side, 332–33
atonic reactions, defined, 24
Aveeno, 101, 231

B
Bach Flower Remedies, 188
back problems, water therapy for, 164–65
bacteria in body
    antibiotic-resistant, 6
    mutations, 6
    natural treatment, 222, 223
bandages, frozen, 23, 45, 224
baths, 67–84. See also footbaths
    drawing, without thermometer, 139,
        140
    effects and uses, 67–68
    types of, 23
    water temperature, 139–40
baths, brush, 71, 73–74
    method, 73–74
    therapeutic uses, 73
baths, cold, 1
    in ancient Rome, 1
baths, cold, full, 68–69
    prolonged, for ill persons, 69
    short, for healthy persons, 68–69
    therapeutic uses, 68
baths, cold mitten massage, 71, 72–73, 145
    method, 72–73
    therapeutic uses, 72
baths, friction, 71–74
    types of, 71–74
baths, herb and medicated, 99–113
    apple cider vinegar, 101
    ascorbic acid bath, 112–13
    bran bath, 109–10
    chamomile bath, 107
    cornstarch, borax, sodium
        bicarbonate, 110
    Epsom salt bath, 110–11

hayflower bath, 104–5
oatmeal bath, 104
oatstraw bath, 106
for perspiration induction, 150
pine bath, 107–8
salt bath, 103
salt massage, 101–2
substances used, 99–101
sulphur bath, 112
baths, hot, full, 70–71
cold compress and, 70, 74, 75
male fertility and, 261
method, 70
prolonged, 71
short, 71
therapeutic uses, 70
baths, salt massage, 71, 101–3
baths, shallow (sitz baths), 74–75
alternate hot and cold, 78
cold, prolonged, 76
cold, short, 75
cool, short, 75–76
hot, prolonged, 77–78
method, 74–75
tepid, prolonged, 77
tepid, short, 76–77
therapeutic uses, 74, 181
baths, sponge, 71
baths, warm
LeBoyer technique, 7
sedating effect of, 7
baths, whirlpool, 78–79, 261
therapeutic uses, 78–79
bedsores, 22
bedwetting
general therapy, 167
water therapy, 166–67
bicarbonate of soda
effects in bathwater, 100, 110
bidet, 135
black eyes, 313–14
bladder, 25, 29, 32
blanket packs, 122–25
dry, 124–25
hot moist, 122–24

blisters, 306
under callus, 306
blisters, foot, 197
blood, effects of heat and cold on,
27–28
blood circulation, water and, 5
blood pressure, high
general therapy, 216–17
water therapy, 216
blood pressure, low, 299
body
strengthening, 146
toughening, 147
body odor
general therapy, 168
water therapy, 167–68
body shampoo, 116–17
body temperature, 21
boils, 283
borax, 100, 110
bottled water, 12, 34, 35
good brands, 36
for infants, 39
marketing of, 12
tests of, 12
bowels, 29
brain, 25, 29, 30
aluminum and, 11
temperature of, 44
bran, effects in bathwater, 100
bran bath, 109–10
method, 109–10
therapeutic uses, 109
Brand Cold Bath technique, 20, 69
breast abscess. See mastitis
breasts, inflamed, 268–70
general therapy, 269
water therapy, 268–69
breath, bad
general therapy, 165
water therapy, 165
breathing
cold double compress for, 56
heat and cold effects on, 27
for relaxation, 251

Breitenbach, R. A., 151
bruises, 306–7
    abrasions, 307
    barked shins, 326–27
    cleat bruises, 310
    contusions, 308
    hematoma, 308
    palm bruise, 307–8
    strawberry bruises, 310–11
bunions, 197–98
buoyancy, water for, 22–23
    techniques, 22–23
burns, healing, 20
    clay for, 155
    techniques, 20
bursitis
    deltoid, 328–29
    general therapy, 168–69
    water therapy, 168
bursitis, knee, 321

C

cabbage leaf poultices, 153, 154, 155,
        156, 160–61
calf cramps, 324–25
calluses, 311
    swimmer's callus, 311
candidiasis (yeast infection), 281
carbon filters, 14, 35
carcinogens, 35
carpal tunnel syndrome
    general therapy, 170
    water therapy, 169–70
castor oil, 154, 160
cayenne pepper, 39, 259
    in footbaths, 90
cell salt therapy, 188, 236
Celsus, 1
chamomile
    bath, 107
    enemas, 22
    tea, 39
Chapman, J. B., 169
charcoal, activated, 155
charley horse, 334–35

chest area
    cold double compress for, 56–57
    criss-cross chest compress, 242–43
    showering, 134
    triangular compress for, 55–56
chest strain (pectoral strain), therapy for,
        312–13
    floating ribs, 312
    solar plexus blow, 313
chickenpox, 283–84
childbirth
    water therapy, 269–70
children
    bad-tasting medicine, 283
    bedwetting therapies, 166, 167, 283
    chronic diarrhea, 181–82
    diseases, 4
    ear infections, 186
    inflammations, 226
    itching in, 231–32
    mouth sores, 236–37
    strengthening, 294–95
    water therapy for, 283–95
chlorine, 11–12, 35
chronic fatigue syndrome
    general therapy, 171
    water therapy, 170–71
clay, 153–56
clay packs, 126–27
clay poultices, 153
clay water, 153
cleansing, 21
clean water, 10–14
    benefits of, 10–11
coffee, for asthma, 163
Coke syrup, 155
cold application
    alternating with heat application to
        same area, therapeutic uses, 28, 32
    to head, 44–45
    prolonged, reflex effects on body
        organs, 30–31
    short, reflex effects on body organs, 29
    therapeutic uses, 19–24, 26–31,
        32–33, 41–45

cold application, effects
    on blood, 27
    on body organs, 24, 26, 29, 30–31
    on heart, 26
    on heat production, 28
    on kidneys, 28
    on lungs, 27
    on metabolism, 27
    on muscles, 27
    on nerves, 26
    on skin, 26
    on stomach, 28
cold baths, 20, 27
cold mitten massage bath, 71, 72–73, 145
colds
    drinking water and, 37
    foot compress for, 63
    general therapy, 172–73
    water therapy, 171–72
cold showers, 129–30, 145–46
    therapeutic uses, 129–30
cold sores
    general therapy, 173–74
    water therapy, 173, 284
cold water. See also baths, cold; com-
        presses, cold
    actions of, 9
    drinking, 2, 5
    fever reduction and, 2
    health uses, 19
    Kneipp and, 3
    therapeutic uses, 9
    tonic techniques, 145–47
    treading in, 5
    walking in, 3
cold-water ankle splash, 147
cold-water friction massage, 243
cold-water treading, 5, 20, 86–87, 146,
        271
    method, 86–87
    therapeutic uses, 86
colic, intestinal, 32
    in children, 284
    hot moist compresses for, 49
collective unconscious, 7

Comfort Corner, 198, 201
comfrey, 154
Commensal, 227
compresses, 47–65. See also packs
    additions to water, 48
    apple cider vinegar, 48, 52
    area, 48
    arnica, 48
    double, 48
    eye, 80
    herb-dipped, 51, 52, 105
    kinds of, and applications, 47
    triangular, 55–56
    witch hazel, 48, 52
compresses, alternate hot and cold, 47
compresses, cold, 2, 9, 20, 23, 47
    hot baths and, 70, 74, 75, 90
    with perspiration induction, 45
compresses, cold double, 47
    body compress, 119–22
    therapeutic uses, 53–54
    throat compress, 54–56
compresses, cold double, abdominal, 58–59
    method of application, 59
    therapeutic uses, 58–59
compresses, cold double, for chest, 56–57
    methods of application, 56–57
    therapeutic uses, 56
compresses, cold double, for foot (wet
        sock), 63
    method of application, 63
    therapeutic uses, 63
compresses, cold double, for genitals,
        61–62
compresses, cold double, for joints, 60
    method of application, 60
    therapeutic uses, 60
compresses, cold double, for trunk, 58
    method of application, 58
    therapeutic uses, 58
compresses, cold single, 47, 51–53
    duration of use, 5 3
    method of application, 52–53
    temperature of, 53
    therapeutic uses, 51–52

compresses, cold single, for foot, 62–63
compresses, cold single, for joints, 60
    method of application, 60
    therapeutic uses, 60
compresses, cold single, for trunk,
        57–58
    method of application, 57–58
    therapeutic uses, 57
compresses, hot, 20, 22, 47
    double, 47
    single, 47
compresses, hot medicated, 51
compresses, hot moist, 23, 49–51
    duration of use, 49
    for hemorrhoids, 61, 62
    for joints, 61
    method of application, 50–51
    sciatica and, 49
    therapeutic uses, 49
compresses, hot single, for foot (wet
        sock), 64
    method, 64
    therapeutic uses, 64
congestion, 32
constipation
    drinking water and, 37
    general therapy, 174–75
    water therapy, 174
contact lens problems, 175
contusions, 308
    charley horse from, 334–35
convulsions, 22
    in children, 285
coughs
    general therapy, 176
    water therapy, 175–76
cramps, 38, 39, 323–24
    muscle therapy, 177
    water therapy, 177
cranberry extract, 233
criss-cross chest compress, 242–43
Crohn's disease, 226–27
crying spells, in children, 285–86
Currier, James, 2
cuts, in children, 286

cystitis, 270–71
    general therapy, 270–71
    water therapy, 270

D

damp sheet packs, 20, 21, 22, 24, 119–22
    cold, 119–22
Dead Sea salts, 101, 103, 246
    effects in bathwater, 100
dehydration, 5, 10, 15
    avoiding effects of, 180
    effects on body, 116–17
    preventing while exercising, 298
dentures, 223
depression
    general therapy, 178
    water therapy, 177–78
detoxification, 5
diabetes
    drinking water and, 37
    general therapy, 179–80
    water therapy, 178–79
diarrhea
    acute, 180–81, 182
    in children, 286
    chronic, 181–82
    clay for, 155
    general therapy, 182
    stopping, 181
digestive aid, 182
digestive problems, 39
    digestive aid, 182
    drinking water and, 38
diphtheria, in children, 286–87
disabled persons, 22
dislocations
    knee, 322–23
    shoulder, 329
Di Stephano, Vincent, 328
distillation, 14
distilled water, 36
diuretic(s), 299
    water as, 21
dizziness, in children, 287
Don't Drink the Water (Lono A'o), 13

dousing shower, 135–36
    method, 136
    therapeutic uses, 135–36
drinking water, 2, 5, 22, 35–39. *See also*
    water intake
    athletes and, 38–39, 298–99
    elderly and, 299
    health problems responding to,
       36–38
    for infants, 39
drop-of-water bath
    method, 82
    therapeutic uses, 82
drugs, and drinking water, 38
dry blanket pack
    method, 125
    therapeutic uses, 124
dry mouth, 184, 237
Duke, James, 185
duodenal ulcers, 184

E
ear bath, 81
ear infections
    general therapy, 185–86
    mastoiditis and, 289–90
    water therapy, 185
ear problems, 185–87
    cold double compress for, 54–56
earth packs, 126–28
    therapeutic uses, 126–27
ear wax, 186
eczema
    general therapy, 187–88
    water therapy, 187
edema, 211
    drinking water and, 37
    effects in bathwater, 100
Effects of Water, Cold and Warm, as a
    Remedy in Fever and Other
    Diseases, The (Currier), 2
Egypt, ancient, 67
elderly persons
    fluid intake, 299
elimination, water therapy, 188–89

eliminative, water as, 21
emetic, water as, 21
enemas, 21, 136–38
    chamomile, 22
    method, 137–38
    therapeutic uses, 136–37
energy flow, restoring with water
    therapy, 4
Epsom salt bath, 21, 110–11, 168
    effects in bathwater, 100, 111
    method, 111
    therapeutic uses, 110–11
eruptions, 288
Evian bottled water, 36, 39
exercise
    preventing dehydration during, 298
    recovery from, 300
expectoration, 31
    expectorant aid, 243–44
eye bath, 80
    method, 80
    therapeutic uses, 80
eye injuries, therapy for, 313–14
eyes
    contact lens problems, 175
    inflamed, 225

F
face
    inflamed, 225
    showering, 135
facial neuralgia, 237
facials, steam, 10, 142
Falkow, Stanley, 6
fatigue
    general therapy, 190
    water therapy, 189–90
feet, 25. *See also* footbaths; foot problems
    Achilles tendon, 300
    calluses, 311
    fractures, 315–16
    heel bruise, 315
    injuries, 315–16
    sole of foot injury, 315
    stiff big toe, 337

feet *continued*
swimmer's callus, 311
toe sprains, 336–37
felons, 97
fennel, effects in bathwater, 100
Fernie, William, 266
fertility, male, and hot baths, 261
fever reduction, 2, 20
Brand Bath for, 69
drinking water and, 5, 37
techniques, 20
water therapy, 190–92
filtered water, 12
carbon filters, 14, 35
finger injuries, 314
Finland, 2
Fitzgerald, William, 164, 172–73, 176, 259
Fiuggi water, 36
Flickstein, Aaron M., 253
flu, 193–96
general therapy, 196
fluid intake
athletes, 38–39, 298, 299
fluoride, 11, 12
fomentations, 47
food poisoning, water therapy, 196–97
footbaths, 85–93
and armbath, simultaneous, 146
therapeutic uses, 85
waterproof bag and, 84
footbaths, alternate hot and cold, 90–91
method, 91
therapeutic uses, 90–91
footbaths, cold, 85
prolonged, 88
running water, short, 87–88
short cold-water treading, 86–87
short shallow toe bath, 87
footbaths, herbal
hayflower, 92, 105–6
oatstraw, 93, 106
footbaths, hot, 21, 85
cold compress to head and, 90
herbal additions to, 90

method and temperature, 89–90
therapeutic uses, 89
footbaths, hot and cold contrast, 90
footbaths, warm
method and temperature, 89
therapeutic uses, 88–89
foot problems, 197–202. *See also* feet;
footbaths
aching, 197
blisters, 197
bunions, 197–98
burning, 198
cold, 198–99
cold single compress for, 62–63
hammertoes, 200–1
odor, 199–200
perspiration (excessive), 201
showering, 132–33
swollen, 201
water therapy and/or general therapy
for, 197–201
friction baths, tonic
brush bath, 73–74
cold mitten massage bath, 72–73
sponge bath, 71–72
friction massage, 21, 23, 33
frostbite
general therapy, 202
water therapy, 201–2
frozen bandages, 23, 45
making, 45
frozen shoulder, 329–30

G
Gaby, Alan, 186, 187–88
Galen, 1
Galland, Leo, 186
gallbladder, 32
water therapy, 202
gallstones, 49
drinking water and, 37
gargles, 255, 259
gastric secretion, 31
gastrointestinal system, 29, 31, 32
genital injuries, therapy for, 316–18

genital irrigation, 21
genitals, cold double compress for, 61–62
German measles, 288
Gilbert, Susan, 299
gingerroot, 51
    in footbaths, 90
    tea, effects in bathwater, 100
gout, 202–3
    general therapy, 203
    water therapy, 203
Greece, ancient, 1, 67
Green Pharmacy (Duke), 185
groin strain, 317–18
groundwater, 10–11
growths, minor, poultices for, 155
gums, 240
    problems, water therapy, 203

H
hair wash. *See* shampoo
hamstring injury, 335–36
hand baths, 95–97
    alternate hot and cold, therapeutic
        uses, 97
    cold, therapeutic uses, 95–96
    hot, therapeutic uses, 96–97
    surgical glove and, 84
hand injuries, therapy for, 318–19
hands, 25
    cramps, 323
    washing, 223
Hanks, John, 113
Hare, H. A., 69
hay fever, 204–5
    water therapy, 204
hayflower, allergy to, water therapy for,
    204
hayflower bath, 104–5, 290–91
    method, 105
    therapeutic uses, 104–5
hayflower compresses, 105
hayflower extract, 93, 96, 97, 105
    effects in bathwater, 100
hayflower footbath, 92
hayflower footbaths, 105–6

hayflower tincture, 104
head, cold application to, 44–45
headaches, 205–8
    causes, 205, 206–7
    circulatory, 207
    functional, 206–7
    organic, 207
    therapy for, 206–7, 208
head baths, 81
    kinds of, 81
    therapeutic uses, 81
healthy persons, full cold baths for,
    68–69
heart, 25, 332
    effects of heat and cold on on,
        26–27
heart problems, 208–211
    acute endocarditis, 210–11
    acute shock, 208–9
    angina, 209–10
    edema, 211
    myocarditis, 210
    water therapy, secondary, 208–11
heart rate, 29, 31
heat, local, 23, 41
heat production, effects of heat and cold
    application on, 28
heat rash, 212–13
heat reactions, 211–13
    heat exhaustion, 211–12
    heat rash (prickly heat), 212–13
    water therapy and general therapy,
        211–13
heatstroke, trigger point for, 212
hematoma, 308–9
    prevention of, 42
hemorrhoids, 231
    ascorbic acid sitz baths for, 113
    general therapy, 214
    hot moist compress for, 62
    water therapy, 213–14, 225
herbal compresses, 51, 52
herbal teas, 21, 39, 68
herbal therapies, and water techniques,
    3–4

hernia
    children's, 289
    hiatus hernia, 217
herpes, 151, 173–74
herpes simplex
    general therapy, 215
    water therapy, 214–15
herpes zoster, 251
hiccups, water therapy, 215
Hippocrates, 1, 67
Hirata, Isao, 335
historical background of water therapy,
    1–4
Hoffman, Ronald L., 183, 226–27
holistic medicine
    elements of, 4
home sauna, 144
home steam bath, 143
    constructing, 143
    therapeutic uses, 143
home treatment systems, 12–14
hot baths, 21, 22, 70–71, 150–51
hot drinks, 298
hot flashes, 271–72
hot packs, 21
hot shower, therapeutic uses, 130
hot tubs, 150–51
    male fertility and, 261
    precautions, 150
    pregnancy and, 278
hot water
    actions of, 9–10
    therapeutic uses, 9–10
hot-water application
    alternating with cold application to
        different area, therapeutic uses,
        28, 32
    alternating with cold application
        to same area, therapeutic uses,
        28, 32
    effects on blood, 28, 41
    effects on body, 24, 26
    effects on heart, 27
    effects on heat production, 28
    effects on kidneys, 28

effects on lungs, 27
effects on metabolism, 27
effects on muscles, 27
effects on nerves, 26
effects on skin, 26
effects on stomach, 28
reflex effects on body functions, 31–32
therapeutic uses, 19–28, 31–33
hot-water bottles, 21, 23, 64–65, 154
    substitutes, 64, 65
    therapeutic uses, 64–65
humidifiers, cool air, 10, 24, 142
Hydrastine (Enzymatic Therapy), 264
hydration, 297–99
hydrotherapy. See water therapy

I
ice, 8, 19
    functions of, 9, 41–42
ice bags, 42, 43, 44
    described, 43
    therapeutic uses, 43
    wrapped, 42
ice hats, 44
ICE (Ice, Compression, Elevation), 42
ice packs, 20, 23, 44
    therapeutic uses, 43–44
ice therapy, 41–45
    length of time, 42
    uses, 9, 41–45
ice turban, making, 44
ice water immersion, 20
immune system, vitamin supplements
    and, 205
incontinence
    general therapy, 218, 219
    water therapy, 217–18
India, 2
indigestion, 183
    acute, 220
    chronic, 221–22
    flatulence, 220–21
    pain, 221
    water therapy and general therapy,
        220–22

infants
    drinking water for, 39
    LeBoyer warm bath technique, 7
infection, 222–23
    general therapy, 223
    water therapy, 223
infections, 28, 32
    general therapy, 223
inflammation, 32
    abscess, 225
    anus, scrotum, prostate, hemorrhoid,
        225
    in children, 226
    external, 224
    eye, 225
    face, 225
    internal deep, 225–26
    mastoiditis, 225
    minor, 224–25
    water therapy, 224–25
    water therapy, by body organ, 228–29
inflammatory bowel disease (IBD),
    226–27
influenza, 193–96
injuries, acute, ice application for, 20,
    41–42
insect bites, 227
intestines, 25, 29
irritable bowel syndrome
    general therapy, 229–30
    water therapy, 227
itching
    in children, 231–32
    general, 230
    rectal, 231
Ivker, Robert S., 252

J
Jacuzzi whirlpool baths, 79
jaw
    temporomandibular disorders, 257
jet lag, 232
    general therapy, 232
    water therapy, 232
Jewish bathhouses, in Dark Ages, 67

jockstrap itch, 319
joints
    cold single compress for, 60
    hot moist compress for, 61

K
Kalenak, A., 335
KDF filtration system, 13, 14
Kegel exercises for incontinence, 218, 219
Kellogg, J. H., 123
Kellogg, William, 5–6
Kenny, Sister, 50
kidneys, 25, 29, 31, 32, 36, 297–98
    dehydration effects on, 16–17
    effects of heat and cold on, 28
    of infants, 39
    stimulation of, 21
    urine production and, 21
kidney stones, 232–34
    general therapy, 234
    water therapy, 233
Kloss, Jethro, 166
knee injuries, therapy for, 319–20
    behind kneecap, 322
    bursitis, 321
    cuts, 322
    dislocations, 322–23
    knee joint inflammation, 323
    snapping extension of knee, 323
    sprains, 320–21
knee showers, 146
Kneipp, Sebastian, 3–4, 163, 166, 190,
    289
knuckle injuries, 318
Kuhn, Dr., 287
Kunzle, Johann, 163

L
laryngitis
    general therapy, 235
    water therapy, 234–35
larynx, 25
laxative, water as, 21
lead
    in tap water, 12

LeBoyer warm bath technique, 7
leg bath, alternate hot and cold, 91–92
leg cramps, 235–36, 324
    general therapy, 235–36
    water therapy, 235
Legionnaire's disease, 151
legs, 25
    aching, water therapy for, 197
lemon balm (melissa), 154, 174, 183
liquid, 8, 9, 19
liver, 25, 28, 29
    dehydration effects on, 16–17
lungs, 25, 29, 241–44
    effects of heat and cold on on, 27

M
magnesium, 234, 235
Maine Chance (spa), 84
massage
    salt, 102
mastitis
    general information, 267–68
    water and herbal therapy,
        268
mastoiditis, 225, 289–90
mattresses, water, 22
measles, 290–91
    general therapy, 291
    water therapy, 290–91
medicine, bad-tasting, 283
men
    fertility and hot baths, 261
    hot baths and, 261
    prostate problems, 261–64
    prostatitis, 261–64
    scrotal cooler, 261
    sexual lassitude, 264–65
    water healing for, 261–66
Meniere's disease
    general therapy, 187
    water therapy, 186–87
menopause
    general therapy, 272
menorrhagia, 274–75

menstrual cramps, 177
menstrual problems, water therapy and
    general therapy
    hot moist compress for, 49
    menstrual spasms, 273–74
    painful period (dysmenorrhea),
        272–74
    premenstrual syndrome (PMS), 273
    profuse period (menorrhagia),
        274–75
    scanty or delayed period (amenor-
        rhea), 276–77
menstrual problems, water therapy and
    general therapy for, 272–77
mental activity. *See* brain
metabolic functions, 10
metabolism
    effects of heat and cold on, 27
Minoans, 67
moist heat, 20
Mountain Valley Water, 36
mouth, dry, 184, 237
mouth sores, 236–37
    general therapy, 236–37
    water therapy, 236
mud packs, 24, 126–27
mumps
    general therapy, 293
    water therapy, 292
muscles, therapy for, 323–26
    atrophied muscles, 325
    cramps, 323–24
    effects of heat and cold, 27, 28
    flabby muscles, 192–93
    muscle spasm, 49
    stiff muscles, 325
    swollen muscles, 325
    torn or strained muscles, 325
mustard pack or plaster, 125–26
    method, 126
    therapeutic uses, 125–26
mustard powder, 90
myocarditis, 210
myrrh, 203, 236

N

nasal congestion, in children, 285
nasal irrigation, 252
nasal mucous membrane, 30
National Resources Defense Council,
    bottled water study, 12
Native Americans, 2, 255
naturopaths, 36
neck
    cold double compress for, 54–56
    stiff, 256
    tension in, 325–26
Neptune's Girdle, 58–59
nerves
    effects of heat and cold on, 26
nervousness, water therapy for, 237
Nespor, Gustav, 243
Neti pot, 252, 253
nettle, 204
    effects in bathwater, 100
neuralgia, 237
neuritis, 238
neuritis pain, 154
neutral shower, therapeutic uses, 130
nightmares, zapping, 293
nightshirt, wet, 4
Norman, N. Philip, 231
nose bath
    method, 82
    therapeutic uses, 81–82
nosebleed
    general therapy, 238–39
    water therapy, 238
nutmeg, effects in bathwater, 100

O

oatmeal bath, 104
    method, 104
    therapeutic uses, 104
oatstraw bath, 100, 106
oatstraw footbath, 93
orchitis, 266
Oscillococcinum, 196
osteomyelitis, 28

Overworked Miracle, The (Ross), 6
ozone home treatment system, 14

P

packs, 24. *See also* compresses
    damp cold sheet pack, 119–22
    defined, 48
    dry blanket pack, 124–25
    earth pack, 126–28
    hot moist pack or hat blanket pack,
        122–24
    mustard pack, 125–26
pain relief, 20
    shoulders, 331
    techniques, 20
    water therapy, 239
paraffin baths, 20, 82–84, 238
    method, 83–84
    therapeutic uses, 82–83
Pellegrino, 36
pelvic congestion, 279
pelvic inflammation, women, 278
pelvic organs, 25, 28
    Kegel exercises, 218, 219
pelvis, 30
penicillin, 6
periodontal disease, 240
peristalsis, 32
Persia, 1
perspiration
    action of, 1–2
    excessive (feet), 201
    during exercise, 298
    menopausal night sweats, 271
perspiration induction, 20, 24, 149–51
    cold compresses and, 45
    full hot bath and, 70
    hot moist packs and, 123
    techniques, 21
    water treatments for, 149–50
pharynx, 25
pine bath, 107–9
    method, 108–9
    therapeutic uses, 107–8

pine extract, 101, 108
    effects in bathwater, 100, 108
pleurisy
    water therapy, 241
    water to flush system, 241–42
pneumonia
    general therapy, 244
    water therapy, 242–44
poison ivy, 244–45
poison oak, 244–45
poison sumac, 244–45
Poland Spring, 36
polio, hot moist compresses for, 50
pollution, 10, 11
pools, 22
potassium, 39
poultices
    cabbage leaf, 153, 154, 155, 156
    clay, 153
    clay and castor oil, for arthritis,
        154
    potato, 156
pregnancy, water therapy, 277–78
Preissnitz, Vincent, 2–3, 124
premenstrual syndrome (PMS), 273
Press, Edward, 150
pressure, 9
prickly heat, 212–13
prostate, 225
prostatitis, 261–64
    acute stage, 262–63
    chronic, 263–64
    pain, 262
    prevention, 262
    therapy for various stages of,
        262–64
pruritis ani, 231
psoriasis
    general therapy, 246–47
    water therapy, 245–46
public tubs or saunas, 151

R

rectal area. *See* anal area
rectal irrigation. *See* enemas

rectum, 32
    compresses for, 61–62
reflex arcs, 8
refrigeration of tap water, 13
rehabilitation, ice therapy for, 41
relaxation, water therapy for, 7, 330–31
respiration, 31
restorative, water as, 19
    techniques, 20
reverse-osmosis systems, 13
Rhazes, 1
rheumatism, drinking water and, 37
RICE (Rest, Ice, Compression,
        Elevation), 239, 331, 333
ringworm, 319
    general therapy, 247
    water therapy, 247
Roberts, William, 299
Rodriguez, Jose, 38–39
Rome, ancient, 1
rosacea
    general therapy, 248
    water therapy, 247–48
rosemary, effects in bathwater, 100
Ross, Sidney, 6
rubella, 288
Russia, 2

S

sage
    effects in bathwater, 100
    gargles, 255
saliva, 184, 237
salt, effects in bathwater, 99
salt bath
    therapeutic uses, 103
salt baths, 20, 21, 22, 103
salt blanket packs, 21
salt intake, athletes and, 38–39
salt massage bath, 71, 101–2, 101–3
    massage, 102
    therapeutic uses, 101–2
salt rubs, 20, 145
salt water, 21
sand packs, hot, 126–27

saunas, 24, 141, 143–44, 150–51
 precautions, 150, 151, 261
 therapeutic uses, 143–44
scarlet fever
 water therapy, 293–94
scars
 general therapy, 249
 water therapy, 248–49
sciatica
 general therapy, 249–50
 hot moist compresses for, 49
 water therapy, 249
Scots shower, 117, 131–32, 145
 therapeutic uses, 132
scrotal cooler, 261
scrotal inflammation, 225
sea salt, 13, 102
sedative, water as, 22
 techniques, 22
self-care, water therapy in, 4
self-healing, 67
sexual lassitude
 general therapy, 265
 in men, 264–64
 water therapy, 264–65
shampoo, 115–17
 for body, 116–17
 for hair, 116
 recommended brands, 116
 therapeutic uses, 115–16
shampoos, 24
Shealy, Norman, 297
sheet bath, 192–93
shingles
 general therapy, 251
 water therapy, 250
shin injuries, therapy for, 326–27
shock, acute, 208–9
shoulder, jet shower to, 134–35
shoulder injuries
 deltoid bursitis, 328–29
 deltoid strain, 328
 frozen shoulder, 329
 loose shoulder, 330
 shoulder dislocation, 329

shoulder separation, 330
 therapy for, 327–31
shoulder pain, water therapy for, 331
showers, 20, 22, 129–36
 alternate hot and cold, 131–32
 bidet, 135
 cold, 129–30, 145–46
 dousing, 135–36
 hot, 130
 knee, 146
 local, 132
 neutral, 130
 Scots, 117, 131–32, 145
 soles of feet, 132–33
 types of, 24
sinus infection
 general therapy, 253–54
 water therapy, 251–53
Sinus Survival (Ivker), 252
sitz bath. *See* baths, shallow
skin
 boils, 283
 effects of heat and cold on on, 26
 elimination through, 20
 eruptions, 288
sleeplessness, 294
smoking, drinking water and, 37
soap, 223
sodium, concentration in blood, 299, 324
sodium bicarbonate, effects in bathwater, 100, 110
sore throat, 254–56. *See also* tonsillitis
 general therapy, 256
 water therapy, 254–56
spermatorrhea (involuntary discharge of semen)
 water therapy, 265–66
sponge bath, 71–72
 method, 72
 therapeutic uses, 71
sponging, 23
sports drinks, 299
sports injuries, 42, 45, 300–37
sprains
 knee, 320–21

sprains *continued*
    toe sprains, 336–37
    water therapy and general therapy,
        300, 309–10, 331–32
Squire, D. L., 298
steam, 8, 19, 24, 141–44
    creating, 10
    therapeutic uses, 10
    vaporizer bath, 141–42
steam room, 150–51
stiff neck, 256
stimulant, water as, 22
    techniques, 22
stitch in side, 332–33
stomach, 25, 30
    effects of heat and cold application, 28
stomach cramps, 182–83
stomach spasms, 183
strains, 310, 325
    bicep strain, 303
    chest strain, 312–13
    deltoid, 328
    elbow strain, 304
    groin strain, 317–18
stupe. *See* compresses, hot medicated
sulphur, 101
    effects in bathwater, 100
sulphur bath, 112
    method, 112
    therapeutic uses, 112
sunstroke, trigger point for, 212
sweat baths, 150–51
swellings
    herbs and clays for, 155–56
Swiss Alpine Hayflower Bath Extract, 105

T
tapeworm, water therapy for, 256–57
tap water, 11–12
    aspirin and, 11
    bottled water and, 36
    filtered, 12, 35
    home treatment system options,
        12–14
    lead in, 12

    running water through, 12
    toxins in, 11–12
teething
    general therapy, 295
    water therapy, 295
temperature of water, 139–40
temporomandibular disorders, 257
tendinitis, therapy for, 333–34
tennis elbow, 304–5
TENS machine, 170
tepid baths, prolonged, 20
testes, rotated, 316
testicles, blows to, 316
testicular inflammation (orchitis)
    water therapy, 266
testicular pain, mumps and, 292
theophylline, in coffee, 163
thigh injuries, 334–36
thirst, 15, 22, 299
throat, 31
    cold double compress for, 54–56
throat compresses, 258–59
thrombus, 327
thymus thump, 190
thyroid, 30, 276
Tiger Balm, 154, 164
tincture of benzoin, 142
toe bath, short cold shallow, 87
toe injuries, 336–37
tonic, water as, 19
tonic reactions, defined, 24
tonic techniques, 20, 145–47
    listed, 145
    to strengthen body, 146
    to toughen body, 147
tonsillitis. *See also* sore throat
    water therapy, 257–59
toxins
    carbon filters and, 35
treading in cold water, 5, 20, 86–87, 146
trunk
    cold double compress for, 58
    cold single compress for, 57–58
Turkeim, Baron, 3
Turkey, 2

U

ulcerative colitis, 226–27
ulcers
    dehydration and, 16
    water therapy, 259–60
urinary tract inflammation, 224
urination
    water intake and, 297–98
    water therapy, 260
uterine hemorrhage, 279
uterine inflammation, 279
uterus, 25, 29, 30, 32

V

vaginal congestion, 280
vaginal douche, 138
    method, 138
    therapeutic uses, 138
vaginal problems, 279–80
vaginal spasms, 280
vaginismus, 281
vaginitis, 279–80
vaporizer bath, 141–42
    method, 142
    therapeutic uses, 141–42
vaporizers, 24, 142
varicose veins, ulcerated, 28
Vitabath, 101
    effects in bathwater, 100
vitamin C, 173–74, 186, 205, 224, 238,
    253
    ascorbic acid bath, 112–13
vitamin supplements, 205
vulva injuries, 317

W

walking, in cold water or wet grass,
    3, 87
warm baths, 22
warm (neutral) water
    actions of, 9
    therapeutic uses, 9
water
    distilled, 36
    drinking water, 2, 5, 22, 35–39

forms of, 8–10
    groundwater, 10–11
water healing. *See* water therapy and
    specific ailments or water
    therapy techniques
water intake. *See also* drinking water
    benefits, 16
    health problems aided by, 36–38
    Robertson's schedule for, 15
    weight and, 15
    for weight loss, 15
water temperature, 139–40
water therapy
    action/reaction effects in body, 88
    benefits of, 4–7
    detoxification by, 5
    direct versus indirect applications
        and effects, 7–8
    as enjoyable, 7
    general effects on body, 24, 25, 26
    health uses, 19–23
    historical background, 1–4
    as holistic medicine, 4–7
    techniques, 19–156
    where to apply for various problem
        areas, 25
weight loss, water intake and, 14–17
Weil, Andrew, 204
Weiss, Rudolf Fritz, 166, 277
whirlpool baths, 20, 78–80, 150–51
    footbaths, 86
    therapeutic uses, 78–79
Whitaker, Julian, 174, 244, 253, 263, 264
Wilson, Erasmus, 3
Winter, Arthur, 170
Winter, Ruth, 170
Winternitz, William, 8
witch hazel compresses, 48
women
    breast abscess (mastitis), 267–68
    cystitis, 270–71
    menopause, 271–72
    menstrual problems, 272–77, 278
    pelvic inflammation, 278–79
    pregnancy, 277–78

women *continued*
    spasms in pelvic area, 278
    vaginal problems, 279–80
    water healing for, 267–81
wrist, sore, 318–19

Y
yogurt, 38, 169

Z
zinc, 188, 253–54
Zone Therapy. *See* Fitzgerald, William
Zorgniotti, Adrian, 261